MOLECULAR ALCHEMY

Unlocking the Therapeutic Power of Hydrogen

New Hope for Cancer and Chronic Diseases, and Strategies to Reverse Aging

MIKE VAN THIELEN, PHD.

Copyright © 2024 Michel Van Thielen ©

All rights reserved.

ISBN: 9798340560766

DEDICATION

This book is for the health heroes who refuse to settle for merely managing symptoms or drowning in a sea of prescriptions and surgeries. It's for those who believe in prevention over treatment and understand that conventional medicine often misses the mark when it comes to tackling root causes.

It's dedicated to the seekers of knowledge about natural and straightforward methods to help the body work its magic and achieve peak health. Here, you'll discover the wonders of molecular hydrogen—a nifty, safe, and easily administered gas with the potential to turn the tables on neurodegenerative diseases, autoimmune disorders, cancer and more. Plus, it's a top contender for boosting longevity and performance for anyone looking for an extra edge.

Don't be just another patient in the conventional medicine conveyor belt; become a savvy explorer of the tiniest molecule on Earth—molecular hydrogen. New hope and the chance to become your best self are just a page away!

NOTE

This book is all about expanding your mind, not your medical or legal liabilities! Consider it a treasure trove of educational gems rather than a substitute for professional advice. While the content is backed by solid scientific research, it's here to enlighten, not to prescribe.

For a full list of studies and scientific articles that make this book's claims more credible than your uncle's fish stories, scan the code:

TABLE OF CONTENTS

DEDICATION
ENDORSEMENTS
ABOUT THE AUTHOR
INTRODUCTION   25

CHAPTER 1:
FROM ALCHEMY TO MODERN MARVEL   28

1.1. EARLY USES AND DEVELOPMENT   29
1.2. H_2 IN INDUSTRY AND ENERGY   29
1.3. HYDROGEN IN THE 21ST CENTURY   30
1.4. CHALLENGES/FUTURE DIRECTIONS   31
1.5. DOES OUR BODY PRODUCE H_2?   32
1.6. MEDICAL APPLICATIONS OF H_2 34

CHAPTER 2:
DECODING H_2 CHEMISTRY   38

2.1. WHAT IS MOLECULAR HYDROGEN?   38
2.2. HYDROGEN CATIONS   39
2.3. HYDROGEN ANIONS   40
2.4. HOW DO THEY COMPARE?   40
2.5. H_2 VS. HYDROGEN PEROXIDE   41

CHAPTER 3:
MOLECULAR HYDROGEN IN ACTION 43

3.1. ANTIOXIDANT PROPERTIES	44
3.2. ANTI-INFLAMMATORY EFFECTS	45
3.3. CYTOPROTECTIVE EFFECTS	47
3.4. ANTI-APOPTOTIC EFFECTS	47
3.5. H_2 AND AUTOPHAGY	48
3.6. METABOLIC REGULATION	50
3.7. IMMUNO-MODULATION	51
3.8. NEUROPROTECTIVE EFFECTS	52
3.9. ANTI-CANCER EFFECTS	52
3.10. H_2 AND SLEEP	52
3.11. H_2 AND PAIN	53

CHAPTER 4:
CANCER AND CHRONIC DISEASES – BATTLING THE BODY'S BIGGEST CHALLENGES 56

4.1. TINY TITAN TAKING ON TUMORS	57
4.1.1. SELECTIVE ANTIOXIDANT	58
4.1.2. ANTI-INFLAMMATORY	59
4.1.3. CELL SIGNALING PATHWAYS	59
4.1.4. BOOSTING CANCER THERAPIES	60
4.1.5. CANCER PREVENTION	62
4.1.6. TYPES OF CANCER	63
4.2. NEURODEGENRATIVE DISEASES	69
4.2.1. SLAYING OXIDATIVE STRESS	70

- 4.2.2. ANTI-INFLAMMATORY PROPERTIES — 70
- 4.2.3. MITOCHONDRIAL PROTECTION — 71
- 4.2.4. INHIBITION OF APOPTOSIS — 71
- 4.2.5. REGULATION OF AUTOPHAGY — 71
- 4.2.6. EXCITOTOXICITY — 72
- 4.2.7. BOOSTING BRAIN POWER — 72
- 4.2.8. BLOOD-BRAIN BARRIER — 73
- 4.2.9. CLINICAL STUDIES — 75

4.3. GI AND DIGESTIVE CONDITIONS — 77
- 4.3.1. H_2 AND ELECTRICAL POTENTIAL — 81
- 4.3.2. GUT MICROBIOTA MODULATION — 83
- 4.3.3. THE GUT GUARDIAN — 83

4.4. METABOLIC DISEASES — 84
- 4.4.1. ANTIOXIDANT ARMOR — 85
- 4.4.2. ANTI-INFLAMMATORY EFFECTS — 85
- 4.4.3. ISULIN SENSITIVITY — 85
- 4.4.4. MITO FUNCTION — 86
- 4.4.5. LIPID METABOLISM — 86
- 4.4.6. BLOOD PRESSURE — 87
- 4.4.7. GUT MICROBIOTA — 87
- 4.4.8. CLINICAL STUDIES — 88

4.5. AUTO-IMMUNE DISEASES — 89
- 4.5.1. ROS RAMPAGE — 89
- 4.5.2. THE CYTOKINE STORM — 90
- 4.5.3. IMMUNE MODULATION — 90
- 4.5.4. TISSUES AND ORGANS — 91
- 4.5.5. MITO PROTECTION — 92
- 4.5.6. CLINICAL STUDIES — 92

4.5.7. THE GUT-IMMUNE LINK	93
4.6. CARDIOVASCULAR DISEASES	**94**
4.6.1. MECHANISMS OF ACTION	95
4.6.2. APPLICATIONS	96
4.7. RESPIRATORY CONDITIONS	**99**
4.7.1. MECHANISMS OF ACTION	99
4.7.2. APPLICATIONS	101

CHAPTER 5:
MASTERING MITOCHONDRIAL HEALTH

	105
5.1. MITO BY NUMBERS	**105**
5.2. THE POWERHOUSE BREAKDOWN	**109**
5.2.1. MITO STRUCTURE	109
5.2.2. MITO SUPERPOWERS	110
5.2.3. MITO DNA	111
5.2.4. MITO DYNAMICS	112
5.2.5. ENERGY PRODUCTION	112
5.3. MITO DYSFUNCTION	**113**
5.3.1. GENETIC FACTORS	114
5.3.2. TOXEMIA EXPLAINED	116
5.3.3. LIFESTYLE MODIFICATIONS	124
5.4. BOOST THE POWERHOUSE	**131**
5.4.1. FIGHT OXIDATIVE STRESS	132
5.4.2. POWER-UP	132

5.4.3. PROTECT DNA	133
5.4.4. BUILD NEW MITO	133
5.4.5. COOL INFLAMMATION	134
5.4.6. MITO MEMBRANE	134
5.4.7. BRAIN POWER	135

CHAPTER 6:
THE ART OF LONGEVITY & RADIANT BEAUTY 137

6.1. IMPACT OF H_2 ON AGING	137
6.1.1. OXIDATIVE STRESS	140
6.1.2. ANTI-INFLAMMATION	140
6.1.3. AGE-RELATED DISEASES	141
6.1.4. SUPPORT MITO FUNCTION	142
6.1.5. CELLULAR REPAIR	142
6.1.6. COGNITIVE FUNCTION	143
6.1.7. TELOMERE PROTECTION	143
6.2. BIOHACKING OUR DNA	146
6.2.1. ARTD1 REPAIR SYSTEM	146
6.2.2. NAD^+ AND NADPH	147
6.2.3. NRF2 PATHWAY	157
6.2.4. MAGNESIUM MAGIC	160
6.2.5. NITRIC OXIDE	163
6.2.6. METHYLENE BLUE	168
6.2.7. THE BUCKY BALL	173
6.2.8. VITAMIN D	177

6.3. THE POWER OF BREATH ... 178
   6.3.1. THE ART OF BREATHING ... 179
   6.3.2. ROLE OF CO_2 TOLERANCE ... 180
   6.3.3. IMPROVING CO_2 TOLERANCE ... 181
   6.3.4. CELLULAR ENERGY ... 183
   6.3.5. BENEFITS FOR MIND/BODY ... 184
   6.3.6. BREATH AND H_2 INHALATION ... 185

6.4. SKIN BEAUTIFICATION AND H_2 ... 186
   6.4.1. OXIDATIVE STRESS ... 189
   6.4.2. INFLAMMATION MITIGATION ... 190
   6.4.3. COLLAGEN PRODUCTION ... 190
   6.4.4. SKIN HYDRATION ... 191
   6.4.5. SKIN REJUVENATION ... 191
   6.4.6. TOPICAL AND SYSTEMIC APPLICATIONS ... 191

CHAPTER 7:
THE NEXT FRONTIER IN ATHLETIC EXCELLENCE ... 194

7.1. THE ANTIOXIDANT ADVANTAGE ... 195
7.2. INFLAMMATION ERASER ... 195
7.3. BOUNCE BACK FASTER ... 196
7.4. POWER-UP ... 196
7.5. FATIGUE FIGHTER ... 197
7.6. MITO MOJO ... 197
7.7. MENTAL CLARITY ... 198
7.8. WHAT SCIENCE SAYS ... 198

CHAPTER 8:
NAVIGATING H₂ PRODUCTS – KEY INFO FOR SAVVY CONSUMERS   201

8.1. HYDROGEN TABLETS   204
8.2. HYDROGEN DEVICES   206
    8.2.1. ELECTROLYSIS MAGIC   206
    8.2.2. PROTON EXCHANGE MEMBRANES   207
8.3. H₂ WATER VS. INHALATION   209
8.4. NOT ALL DEVICES ARE CREATED EQUALLY   214
    8.4.1. HYDROGEN CATALYSTS   214
    8.4.2. QUALITY CONSIDERATIONS   214
    8.4.3. COST CONSIDERATIONS   216
8.5. SAFETY AND DOSING – THE LOWDOWN   218

REFERENCES / SCIENTIFIC LITERATURE   224

ENDORSEMENTS

"As a neurologist leading a large practice that integrates wellness modalities, we consistently strive for cutting-edge treatments to improve patient outcomes. One of the most transformative additions to our practice has been molecular hydrogen therapy, which has yielded remarkable results for our patients. So much so, that we have initiated a research program to further assess its efficacy.

Dr. Mike's book, *Molecular Alchemy*, is a comprehensive, science-based resource that beautifully bridges rigorous research with accessible, reader-friendly content. Dr. Mike, a true pioneer in the wellness and biohacking fields, offers a wealth of scientific data while ensuring the material is easily digestible. This book is indispensable for anyone seeking to overcome chronic illness or optimize their physical and mental well-being. *Molecular Alchemy* is a must-read for those on a journey toward better health and longevity."

Dr. Syed Asad, MD, Neurologist
Universal Neurologic Care

"When it comes to biohacking your health, Dr. Mike is simply the best! *Molecular Alchemy* showcases what might be the greatest science-based breakthrough in non-conventional medicine. The therapeutic power of molecular hydrogen, as detailed in this book, holds the key to looking, feeling, and living at your highest potential.

This is an absolute must-read for anyone serious about optimizing their well-being. Dr. Mike's work is transformative, and *Molecular Alchemy* is his latest gift to those ready to unlock their true health potential."

Dr. Fab Mancini
International Bestselling Author and Speaker, Wellness Revolutionaries Hall of Famer

"Dr. Mike Van Thielen, PhD, has done a remarkable job of providing readers with an insightful overview of the myriad health benefits of molecular hydrogen. I'm not aware of any other resource that is both as concise and as comprehensive in explaining how molecular hydrogen can optimize human biology.

Molecular Alchemy offers a unique blend of clarity and depth, making it an essential read for anyone interested in cutting-edge health optimization."

Dr. Jeffrey Gladden, MD, FACC
CEO/Founder/Chief Medical Officer, Gladden Longevity

"As a radiation oncologist with a distinguished career at Mount Sinai in New York City, multiple published articles on cancer, and the establishment of various cancer centers nationwide, I have seen firsthand the positive impact of molecular hydrogen on cancer and other diseases.

Despite common belief that cancer rates are on the rise, emerging scientific research suggests that molecular hydrogen could be a game-changer. Understanding how to harness this novel therapeutic gas to protect against oxidative stress and DNA damage is crucial. This book is an essential read, offering new hope for those battling cancer and chronic illnesses."

V. Rao Emandi, MD, FACRO
Radiation Oncologist

"I've had the pleasure of knowing Dr. Mike Van Thielen, PhD, for over a decade, and I first encountered his passion and expertise in natural medicine and holistic health through our close collaborations and his engaging community lectures.

Dr. Van Thielen is a masterful speaker on a wide range of holistic health topics, a skill vividly showcased in his acclaimed 2014 manuscript, *Health 4 Life*. His deep commitment to preventive medicine and lifestyle management stands in stark contrast to the traditional Western approach of addressing diseases after they arise.

His latest book on molecular hydrogen arrives at a crucial time, offering valuable insights into maintaining long-term health. I wholeheartedly recommend this book to anyone eager to embrace a healthier, more vibrant life."

Dr. Jeffrey Allyn Ruterbusch
Commander, United States Navy (retired)
Aerospace Physiologist/Flight Surgeon
Hyperbaric Medical Officer
Associate Professor, College of Graduate Studies,
Central Michigan University, Mt. Pleasant, Michigan 48859

Board-certified Age-Management Medicine
Board-certified General/Sports Nutrition
Board-certified Integrative Medicine
Board-certified Anti-aging Sports Medicine
Board-certified Functional Medicine
Board-certified, Managed Care Medicine
Diplomate, Sports Nutrition
DO, NMD, MPH, MSA, MS, MS, DACBN, DAAIM, CNS, CSCS, CISSN, CMCM, PAHM, Dip. S.N.
Faculty, Preventive Medicine, Nutrition, and Sports Medicine, Fitness Institute of Technology, Tampa, Florida.

"As the CEO of Biohackers Magazine, I've had the distinct pleasure of collaborating with Dr. Mike Van Thielen for many years. His expertise in holistic health and natural medicine is truly unparalleled. Mike is a trailblazer in the world of health optimization, always pushing the boundaries of what's possible in preventative care. His visionary insights, coupled with his unique ability to distill complex scientific concepts into practical advice, make him an invaluable authority in the wellness community.

Mike's passion for improving lives shines through in every aspect of his work, from his dynamic lectures to his thought-provoking writings. His latest book on molecular hydrogen is no different. It offers a groundbreaking exploration of the health benefits of molecular hydrogen, providing cutting-edge research and practical applications for those looking to elevate their well-being and longevity.

I wholeheartedly recommend this book to anyone committed to optimizing their health. Dr. Mike Van Thielen's contributions to the field continue to shape the future of wellness, and this work only solidifies his status as a leader in the health and wellness space."

Jean Fallacara
CEO, Biohackers Magazine

"As a licensed chiropractor, functional neurologist, and functional medicine practitioner, I've witnessed countless health trends come and go. But occasionally, something truly groundbreaking emerges. *Molecular Alchemy: Unlocking the Therapeutic Power of Hydrogen* is one of those rare game-changers. This book delves into the fascinating science of molecular hydrogen—a molecule so small it makes everything else look bulky!

Dr. Mike Van Thielen's fresh, engaging style makes complex science not only easy to grasp but genuinely enjoyable to read. With a perfect blend of cutting-edge research and practical insights, he reveals why hydrogen could very well be the next frontier in health optimization. Whether you're serious about wellness or just want to impress at dinner parties, this book is must-read.

As someone who's been in the trenches of health optimization for years, I'm throwing on my hydrogen-powered cape and joining the revolution. Thank you, Mike, for sharing this with the world—it's time everyone knew about the incredible potential of hydrogen!"

Dr. Bill Janeshak
Yorbalinda family chiropractic, #1 Chiropractic and Integrated Medicine Clinic in Orange County, California in 2023. Dr. Janeshak received the Presidential Award for Lifetime Achievement in 2024.

"Dr. Mike is consistently ahead of the curve in health and wellness. In this book, he reveals the multitude of benefits and preventative powers of molecular hydrogen.

I highly recommend this book to anyone interested in cutting-edge health innovations. As a chiropractic physician with 25 years of experience, I've gained valuable new insights into achieving optimal wellness. Dr. Mike is truly spot on!"

Robert Devincentis, DC
Intracoastal Chiropractic Clinic, Jacksonville, FL.

"When it comes to biohacking and diving deep into science, Dr. Mike is unmatched! This book is an absolute eye-opener and a must-read for anyone looking to enhance or maintain a healthy lifestyle. But even more importantly, it's essential reading for health care practitioners who want to truly understand and address the root causes of disease.

Dr. Mike breaks it all down—from cancer prevention to innovative beauty tips that literally help you age in reverse. I had the privilege of podcasting with him last year, and his knowledge and experience in health and wellness are nothing short of extraordinary.

As a like-minded practitioner, Dr. Mike transcends the outdated "sick care" model that dominates modern healthcare. He's a true pioneer and educator, guiding us to think beyond the traditional Western approach and toward a future of proactive, holistic health."

Dr. Kourtney Chichilitti, PharmD
Integrative Health Pharmacist
Certified Functional Medicine Practitioner

"Dr. Mike has once again delivered an insightful and groundbreaking book on health. In this work, he skillfully demystifies the science of Molecular Hydrogen, offering a clear and comprehensive explanation of how this tiny molecule can have such a profound impact on our physiology. I particularly appreciate how he substantiates his claims with extensive scientific research and peer-reviewed studies.

As a Biological Dentist with Naturopathic training, I've incorporated medical Ozone into my practice for over a decade, recognizing its numerous biological benefits despite its limited use in conventional medicine. Similarly, Molecular Hydrogen has long been on my radar, but after reading Dr. Mike's book, I'm now fully convinced of its potential.

I'm excited to take the next step by investing in a machine that produces both Molecular Hydrogen gas and water.

Kudos to Dr. Mike for sharing this cutting-edge information, empowering people to achieve better health in a natural, scientifically backed way. This book is a must-read for anyone looking to enhance their well-being."

Chris Edwards, DDS, ND
SMILE Design & Wellness Center

"Fasten your holistic health seatbelts! Dr. Mike has once again knocked it out of the park with his latest book, *Molecular Alchemy*. As a holistic practitioner with 47 years of experience and having had the privilege of collaborating with Dr. Mike for 25 of those years, I can confidently say that his approach to health mirrors the same qualities that led him to break multiple world records in Master's Swimming: dedication, focus, deep knowledge, and unwavering commitment.

Molecular Alchemy embodies all these traits, providing a visionary guide that will elevate both your health and your life to new heights. This book offers not just information but a blueprint for transforming your well-being on a profound level. Read it, absorb its wisdom, and let it transform your life!"

Dr. Jo Dee Baer, PhD
Certified Health Coach
Holistic Nutritionist PhD.

"Dr. Mike Van Thielen has expertly unraveled the complexities of molecular hydrogen, positioning it as the next breakthrough in both preventive and therapeutic health care. As a nurse practitioner specializing in integrative medicine, I am continually impressed by the thorough research and real-world applications presented in this book.

Dr. Mike's groundbreaking insights into how H_2 can address chronic diseases, promote longevity, and enhance athletic performance are truly remarkable. This is a must-read for anyone committed to advancing their health with innovative, science-backed strategies."

Brittany Korell, FNP-C
Integrative Medicine Provider, Panorama Health Integrative Medicine

"Dr. Van Thielen stands out as one of the most dedicated and visionary professionals I've had the privilege to work with. His passion for wellness and anti-aging extends far beyond his extensive knowledge—it's driven by a deep commitment to truly improving the lives of those he serves. What sets him apart is not only his expertise but also the genuine care and compassion he brings to every interaction. He is wholeheartedly devoted to helping others achieve their healthiest, most vibrant selves. I trust and admire him immensely, both as a colleague and as a friend."

Dan Bricker
Wellness Director
Research Project Manager
Universal Neurological Care

"Dr. Mike Van Thielen is a remarkable professional, blending integrity, ingenuity, intelligence, and a steadfast commitment to excellence. Our relationship spans various roles: from being my mentor in nutrition and regenerative medicine to training him to break world and national swimming records, and finally, to enjoying life as friends. Dr. Mike excels as a father, a fierce competitor, and a high achiever.

His latest book on Molecular Hydrogen is an essential read for anyone aiming to stay healthy and reach their peak performance. As a trainer, I've successfully used molecular hydrogen inhalation and hydrogen-infused water to help clients and athletes recover from injuries and perform at their best. It's an honor and a pleasure to be both Dr. Mike's strength trainer and friend."

Tasso C. Kiriakes, MS.
Founder of Bodez Personalized Fitness.
Trainer of National Champions in wrestling, football (NFL), basketball, swimming, baseball (MLB), racquetball, track and field, lacrosse, and NASCAR Hall of Famers / current drivers.

"*Molecular Alchemy* provides a deep dive into one of the most exciting and emerging areas of health and wellness research. The concept of hydrogen as a therapeutic agent is not entirely new, but this book manages to unpack the science behind it in an accessible way, without oversimplifying the complexities involved. Dr. Mike takes readers through the various benefits of molecular hydrogen (H_2), its anti-inflammatory properties, antioxidant potential, and even its neuroprotective effects. What stands out most, however, is the balance between scientific rigor and readability.

The information, though rooted in dense molecular biology and chemistry, is presented in such a way that even readers without a deep scientific background can grasp the fundamental concepts. The author uses helpful analogies and practical examples that make difficult sections easier to digest.

Personally, I was particularly drawn to the chapter discussing molecular hydrogen's role in improving sleep. My own journey with poor sleep had been a frustrating one until I decided to try hydrogen inhalation. After incorporating molecular hydrogen into my nightly routine, I noticed significant improvements. My sleep patterns became more consistent, and even if I woke up briefly during the night I could go back to sleep and wake in the morning feeling rested.

Jo Ellen Kleinhenz, PTA

"It is with great enthusiasm that I offer my full support of Dr. Mike Van Thielen, PhD. I had the honor of meeting Dr. Mike through my esteemed colleague, Dr. Fabrizio Mancini, and I can confidently say that Dr. Mike is an exceptional individual, truly a standout in the field of alternative medicine and holistic health.

Beyond being a world record holder in swimming and a remarkable physical specimen, Dr. Mike is a compassionate, authentic, and deeply caring human being. His vast qualifications—ranging from a PhD in Holistic Nutrition to licenses in physical therapy and acupuncture, along with certifications in numerous therapeutic modalities—are a testament to his unwavering commitment to comprehensive and integrative health care.

What truly distinguishes Dr. Mike is his passion for education and his relentless dedication to helping others. In a field often overwhelmed by fads and unsupported claims, Dr. Mike's approach is a breath of fresh air, rooted firmly in transparency, scientific rigor, and evidence-based practices. His dedication to truth-seeking and his commitment to integrity shine through in all aspects of his work and publications.

Dr. Mike Van Thielen's mission to push the boundaries of alternative medicine and holistic health is both inspiring and impactful.

His unique blend of expertise, passion, and ethical commitment makes him an invaluable asset to the medical community and to anyone seeking optimal health.

I am honored to endorse not only Dr. Mike's latest groundbreaking book but also Dr. Mike himself, as both a professional and an individual. His contributions to holistic health are profound, and I have no doubt his continued work will transform countless lives.

It is with the utmost respect and enthusiasm that I offer my support and admiration for Dr. Mike Van Thielen, a true leader and innovator in the pursuit of health and wellness."

Roberto Beteta Jr.
CEO & Founder of TITN (TransitionITnow.com)
CEO & Founder of BrainWave MedTech Group (Brainwavemtg.com)
Master Distributor and Strategic Partner, WAVimed.com
Strategic Partner and Lead Consultant, HueLightUSA.com

"Dr. Van Thielen is my go-to health guy. Whenever I or my loved ones have a health concern, he's the first person I turn to for advice. His deep knowledge and experience with the human body are truly remarkable. His new book has finally clarified all the buzz about hydrogen for me. I'm now implementing these preventative strategies for my family, especially for my young daughter."

Charlie Williams
CEO World Sports Alumni
Former #1 World Billiards

ABOUT THE AUTHOR...

If Tony Robbins, Elon Musk, and Evander Holyfield had a love child, it would be me. That's because I'm part motivational speaker with a passion for helping others, part innovator driven by big ideas, and part ass-kicker—served with a side of humor and charisma. At least, that's what they say.

Born and raised in Belgium with little more than passion, persistence, a big dream, and two pairs of speedos, I've swum my way to a World Record, lived the American Dream, and become a recognized expert in biohacking and peak performance.

I'm Dr. Mike Van Thielen, Ph.D. in holistic nutrition, physician, mentor, and biohacking expert with over three decades of experience in optimal health, anti-aging, regenerative medicine, sports performance, nutrition, and supplementation. As a top swimmer in my native Belgium, I developed an interest in maximizing health and athletic performance. I graduated from the University of Brussels with a bachelor's in physical education in 1993 and a master's in physical therapy in 1995, later serving as an assistant coach and physical therapist for the Belgian Olympic swimmers at the 1996 Atlanta Games.

After moving to Florida in 1997, I managed several pain management clinics and earned my Master of Science in Oriental Medicine and Bachelor of Science in professional health studies from the Florida College of Integrative Medicine. I am a licensed physical therapist, licensed acupuncture physician, and doctor of Oriental Medicine with certifications in injection therapy, homeopathy, Chinese herbal medicine, and non-invasive cosmetic procedures. I also hold a Ph.D. in Holistic Nutrition from the College of Natural Health. More recently, I obtained certification in Molecular Hydrogen from the Molecular Hydrogen Institute (MHI).

Beyond health, I'm well-versed in business, with multiple certifications and a proven track record of establishing successful ventures. My Corporate Impact program helps businesses improve culture, engagement, and productivity while upgrading employees' bodies and minds. I've owned several anti-aging clinics in Florida, developing systems that retained over 90% of clients and boosted referrals.

In 2008, I founded a company that certified over 1,000 healthcare professionals in wellness, weight loss, and non-invasive cosmetic procedures before selling it in 2014. From 2015 until 2019 when the pandemic started, I was the CEO of a well-recognized stem cell company. We successfully treated 1000's of patients, including top athletes, NFL players and heavy weight boxing champions.

I've written several books, including "Health 4 Life – User Manual", the Amazon bestseller "EMR – The Invisible Threat", and "The IZOD Method™ – Unleash Your Superpower". The IZOD Method™ has been featured on over 300 news channels, including Fox, ABC, NBC, and google news. I'm featured on the cover of Biohackers Magazine, issue 22 and I'm an Executive Contributor for Brainz Magazine. I was presented with the CREA GLOBAL AWARDS 2023 honoree in recognition of my creative and innovative ideas, adaptability in business, and for my contributions to sustainability and mental health projects.

Over the years, I've had the opportunity to encourage and inspire thousands of people across the U.S., Canada and Europe. I'm an international keynote speaker and a TEDx Speaker and I'm featured in Motivational Speakers America alongside Les Brown and

Brian Tracy. I shared the stage with many celebrities including Nick Vujicic, Gary Brecka, Dr. Fab Mancini, Dr. Mercola, Del Bigtree, Darren Hardy, Mirela Sula, David Meltzer, JJ Virgin, Christopher Palmer, Tim Gray, and many more.

As a 2-time All-American and World Record Holder in swimming, with 31 U.S. National Titles and 2 YMCA National Records, I'm a proud member of the World Sports Alumni. Currently, I own Biohacking Unlimited. In between biohacking, mentoring, and entrepreneurship, I'm a proud father of two beautiful daughters and I love traveling and outdoor activities.

Dr. Mike Van Thielen, PhD.

INTRODUCTION

Welcome to the World of Molecular Hydrogen - The Tiny Titan of Health

Imagine a molecule so minuscule it makes a grain of sand look like a skyscraper. That's molecular hydrogen (H_2) for you—the lightest, most abundant element in the universe, now making waves as a medical marvel. Imagine having a superhero in your wellness toolkit, one that's not only super tiny but also super mighty in optimizing your health.

Molecular hydrogen isn't just a laboratory curiosity; it's a game-changer for modern medicine. Thanks to its minute size, it can sneak into every nook and cranny of our cells, offering benefits that larger molecules can only dream of. Whether you're dealing with degenerative diseases like cancer or neurodegenerative disorders, or just trying to fend off the effects of aging, this gas packs a punch. It's got the power to tackle inflammation and oxidative stress—two of the biggest troublemakers in our health.

This isn't just hype; over 2,400 scientific studies back up the impressive claims about molecular hydrogen. It's shown to combat over 170 common ailments, from chronic inflammation to metabolic issues. And get this: its ability to slip through cell membranes and the blood-brain barrier means it can access parts of your body that other antioxidants can't. It's like having a VIP pass to your cellular health party.

Hydrogen's talents don't stop there. It helps manage telomere attrition (keeping your chromosomes in check), influences mitochondrial function, and even improves your gut biome and sleep quality. It's like giving your body a tune-up, with benefits you can enjoy from the comfort of your home.

Want to dive into the science behind this tiny titan? Check out the wealth of studies available on PubMed, Google Scholar, and other research sites. For a deep dive into references and scientific studies mentioned here, just visit the resources page on my website MVTonline.com and select "molecular hydrogen" from the drop-down box.

So, buckle up and get ready to explore how this humble molecule could revolutionize your health and wellness. It's not just a little gas; it's a big deal in the world of medicine!

MOLECULAR HYDOGEN – NEW HOPE

CHAPTER 1
FROM ALCHEMY TO MODERN MARVEL

Hydrogen, the most abundant element in the universe has a rich history that traces back to the dawn of modern chemistry. The name "hydrogen" comes from the Greek words "hydro," meaning water, and "genes," meaning creator—because it forms water when burned. While hydrogen was known in a rudimentary form in the 16th century, it wasn't until the 18th century that scientists recognized it as a distinct element.

The journey began with Paracelsus, a Swiss alchemist in the 16th century, who observed a flammable gas produced when metals were dissolved in acids. However, he didn't identify this gas as an element. In the 17th century, Robert Boyle, an Anglo-Irish natural philosopher, made further advances by studying this gas, calling it "inflammable air." The breakthrough came in 1766 with Henry Cavendish, a British scientist who identified hydrogen as a separate substance. His experiments showed that hydrogen, when burned, produced water, leading him to call it "inflammable air." This discovery set the stage for Antoine Lavoisier, who confirmed that water is composed of hydrogen and oxygen, naming the gas "hydrogen."

1.1. Early Uses and Development

Initially, hydrogen's uses were limited to scientific experimentation. Cavendish's pioneering work laid the groundwork for understanding chemical reactions and elements. However, practical applications didn't emerge until Jacques Charles, in 1783, developed the hydrogen balloon. This innovation marked hydrogen's entry into aeronautics, with its lightweight nature making it ideal for lifting balloons. Hydrogen's role in airships continued into the 20th century, with the infamous Hindenburg being a notable example.

1.2. Hydrogen in Industry and Energy

The 19th century saw hydrogen's industrial applications begin to unfold. A breakthrough came with the Haber-Bosch process in the early 20th century, which synthesizes ammonia from nitrogen and hydrogen. This method revolutionized agriculture by enabling mass production of fertilizers, thus supporting global food production.

As the 20th century progressed, hydrogen found new applications in petroleum refining, where it helps remove sulfur and impurities from crude oil, producing cleaner fuels. Hydrogen's potential as a fuel was recognized as early as 1920, but it wasn't until the space age that it truly shined. During the mid-20th century, hydrogen became a crucial component of rocket fuel, used extensively by NASA in the Apollo missions.

1.3. Hydrogen in the 21st Century

Energy and Beyond

Today, hydrogen is at the cutting edge of sustainable energy discussions. It's a clean-burning fuel, with water being its only byproduct when used.

Hydrogen fuel cells, which convert hydrogen into electricity through a chemical reaction, are being developed for various uses, from powering vehicles to energizing buildings. Investments in hydrogen infrastructure, including refueling stations and production facilities, are driving the adoption of hydrogen-powered vehicles.

Moreover, hydrogen is emerging as a solution for storing energy from renewable sources like wind and solar. This is crucial for balancing energy supply and demand, as

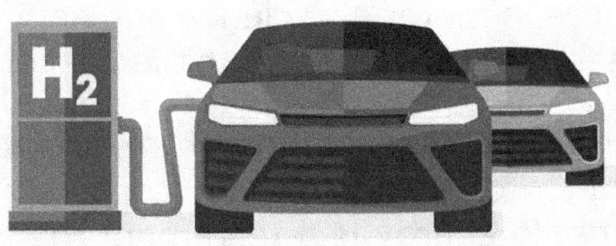

hydrogen can be produced and stored during times of high renewable energy production and used when it's low. Hydrogen is also being explored in industrial processes like steelmaking, where it can replace carbon as a reducing agent, potentially lowering the carbon footprint of steel production.

1.4. Challenges and Future Directions

Despite its promise, hydrogen faces significant hurdles, particularly in production, storage, and distribution. Currently, most hydrogen is produced from natural gas, releasing carbon dioxide in the process. However, there are ongoing efforts to develop "green hydrogen," which is produced from water using renewable energy sources, thereby eliminating these emissions.

Storing and transporting hydrogen is also challenging due to its low density and the high energy required to liquefy or compress it. Advances in materials science and engineering are essential to overcome these challenges.

Hydrogen's evolution from a laboratory curiosity to a potential cornerstone of sustainable energy is a testament to scientific and technological progress. As research and innovation continue, hydrogen's role in the global energy landscape is set to expand, contributing to a cleaner, more sustainable world.

1.5. Does our body produce hydrogen?

Surprise! Our bodies do indeed produce hydrogen, but not quite in the way you might think. Hydrogen is naturally generated through the fermentation of fibers from fruits and veggies by our gut bacteria. Hydrogen is then carried to our cells by our blood plasma. Hydrogen saturation in our blood occurs at 1.8-2.2cc/liter. Excess hydrogen is simply exhaled.

However, if your diet is less than stellar, your digestion is a bit sluggish, or you're just aging (thanks, time!), your hydrogen levels might drop, impacting your cellular and biochemical processes.

How It Works: Our gut is like a bustling metropolis for microbes, including bacteria, archaea, and yeast. These little guys feast on dietary fibers and carbohydrates that our small intestine can't fully digest. During their fermentation party, they produce hydrogen gas among other byproducts. This fermentation mostly happens in the colon where microbial action is at its peak.

- **Fermentation Fiesta:** In the colon, complex carbs and fibers break down into short-chain fatty acids, gases (like hydrogen, methane, and carbon dioxide), and other goodies.
- **Hydrogen Hotspot:** Bacteria from the Firmicutes and Bacteroidetes phyla and certain archaea, like Methanogens, are the stars of this hydrogen production show. They turn dietary fibers and certain sugars into hydrogen.

Why We Need It:

- **Digestive Duty:** Hydrogen is a natural byproduct of your gut's fermentation

process, helping with digestion and metabolic activities.
- **Gut Health Guru:** The production and balance of hydrogen and other gases can affect your gut health and microbiota composition.

Health Implications:

- **Digestive Health:** Normal hydrogen production and excretion are part of healthy digestion. However, too much or too little can lead to bloating and gas.
- **Metabolic Magic:** While gut-produced hydrogen is not the same as therapeutic hydrogen (like from hydrogen-rich water or inhalation), it might still impact your overall health and metabolic processes.

In summary, your body makes hydrogen mainly through gut fermentation, contributing to digestion and overall gut health. This hydrogen gets absorbed into the bloodstream and exhaled. While this natural production is part of normal function, researchers are exploring its potential health benefits.

1.6. Medical Applications of Hydrogen

Recently, hydrogen has garnered attention for its potential medical benefits, particularly due to its antioxidant properties.

Molecular hydrogen (H_2) has been found to selectively neutralize harmful reactive oxygen species (ROS) in the body, which are linked to various diseases and aging processes. This makes hydrogen a promising candidate for treating conditions caused by oxidative stress, including neurodegenerative diseases like Parkinson's and Alzheimer's, cardiovascular diseases, and certain cancers.

Hydrogen therapy can be administered in several ways: through hydrogen-rich water, inhalation of hydrogen gas, or hydrogen-rich saline injections. Studies show that consuming hydrogen-rich water can improve symptoms in patients with conditions such as metabolic syndrome, rheumatoid arthritis, and diabetes. Inhalation of hydrogen gas, which allows for rapid absorption, has shown potential in reducing brain injury severity, protecting the heart during cardiac procedures, and improving stroke outcomes.

Another exciting area of research is hydrogen's role in preventing and treating radiation-induced damage, especially relevant in cancer therapy. Hydrogen's ability to reduce oxidative stress and inflammation may help protect healthy tissues from the harmful effects of radiation, potentially leading to more effective and less damaging cancer treatments.

Despite the promising evidence, more research is needed to fully understand hydrogen's mechanisms, optimal delivery methods, and long-term effects. Ongoing clinical trials aim to validate hydrogen therapy's efficacy across various medical conditions, and these results could pave the way for broader adoption of hydrogen in modern medicine.

MOLECULAR HYDOGEN – NEW HOPE

CHAPTER 2

DECODING H_2 CHEMISTRY

Before we dive deeper, let's clarify a key point: **only molecular hydrogen (H_2)** provides the therapeutic benefits we're talking about. Other forms of hydrogen won't give you the same results, so don't be misled by similar-sounding terms.

2.1. What Is Molecular Hydrogen (H_2)?

Molecular hydrogen (H_2) is the smallest and most abundant molecule in the universe. It's made of two hydrogen atoms bonded together, sharing their single electrons. This simple duo is colorless, odorless, non-toxic, but highly flammable. The bond between these atoms is strong, meaning you need a lot of energy to break them apart.

Though H_2 is stable under normal conditions, it can become reactive when exposed to high temperatures or certain catalysts. For example, when hydrogen reacts with oxygen, you get water—and a lot of energy in the process (think explosions and rocket fuel!).

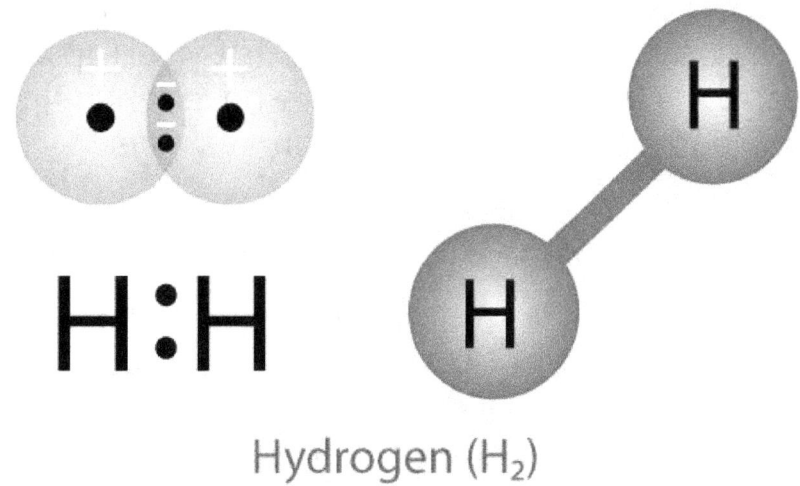

Hydrogen (H_2)

2.2. Hydrogen Cations: Protons (H^+)

When hydrogen loses its electron, it becomes a positively charged ion, known as a proton (H^+). This little proton doesn't float around on its own but bonds with other molecules, like water, to form hydronium ions (H_3O^+). This chemistry is the basis of acids and plays a key role in our body, especially in how cells produce energy.

2.3. Hydrogen Anions: Hydride (H⁻)

On the flip side, if a hydrogen atom gains an extra electron, it becomes a negatively charged hydride ion (H⁻). Hydrides are super useful in chemistry because they donate electrons to other molecules, making them great at reducing reactions. They're found in certain chemical processes and even help in our body's energy production systems.

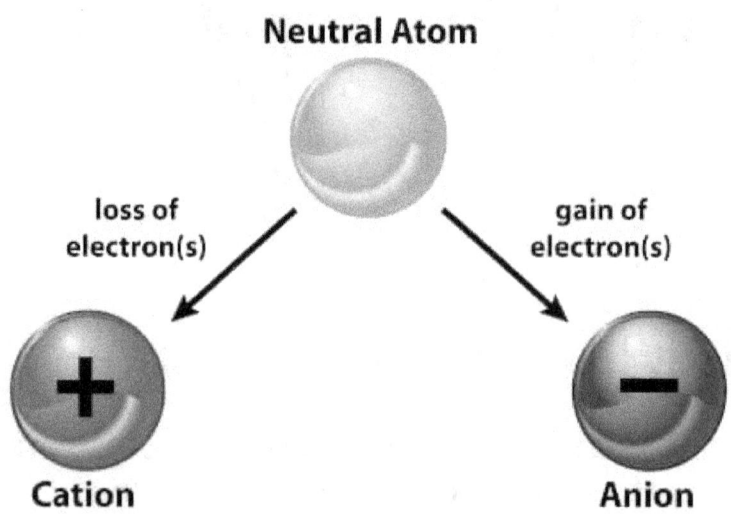

2.4. How Do They Compare?

Molecular hydrogen (H_2) is chill and stable, while its charged cousins, H⁺ and H⁻, are much more reactive. H⁺ (the proton) is essential in acid-base reactions and energy production in our cells, while H^- (the hydride) is a strong reducing agent that's useful in industrial and biological processes. So, while molecular hydrogen is relatively calm, its charged forms bring a lot of chemistry to the table.

2.5. Molecular Hydrogen vs. Hydrogen Peroxide (H_2O_2)

Don't confuse H_2 with hydrogen peroxide (H_2O_2)! They might both have hydrogen, but their roles are very different. H_2 is stable and acts as a reducing agent, while H_2O_2 is unstable, breaks down quickly, and is a strong oxidizer used in disinfecting and bleaching. In terms of safety, hydrogen peroxide can cause burns, while hydrogen gas, though non-toxic, is flammable and needs careful handling.

To sum up, when we talk about hydrogen's benefits in this book, we're referring to molecular hydrogen (H_2)—the form with the real therapeutic effects.

MOLECULAR HYDOGEN – NEW HOPE

CHAPTER 3

MOLECULAR HYDROGEN IN ACTION

Molecular Hydrogen - Unveiling Its Hidden Potential

Molecular hydrogen (H_2) may sound like a topic from a chemistry lecture, but this humble molecule is emerging as a powerhouse in medical science. Traditionally recognized for its roles in industrial applications and as a potential clean energy source, H_2 is now making waves in the realm of health and wellness. This chapter delves into the remarkable physiological effects of molecular hydrogen, exploring its potential in disease prevention and therapeutic applications.

The Power of Molecular Hydrogen

At first glance, molecular hydrogen—a molecule consisting of just two hydrogen atoms—might seem unimpressive. Yet, its simplicity is precisely what makes it so versatile. As the smallest and lightest element in the universe, hydrogen can diffuse rapidly across cell membranes and tissues, enabling it to exert profound effects on a cellular level. Unlike conventional antioxidants that primarily act in specific areas, H_2 can penetrate deeply into cells and mitochondria, providing widespread protective and therapeutic benefits.

3.1. Antioxidant Properties

Molecular hydrogen's most celebrated feature is its role as a selective antioxidant. Antioxidants are crucial for neutralizing harmful reactive oxygen species (ROS) that contribute to oxidative stress—a condition linked to aging, cancer, cardiovascular diseases, and neurodegenerative disorders.

OXIDATIVE STRESS

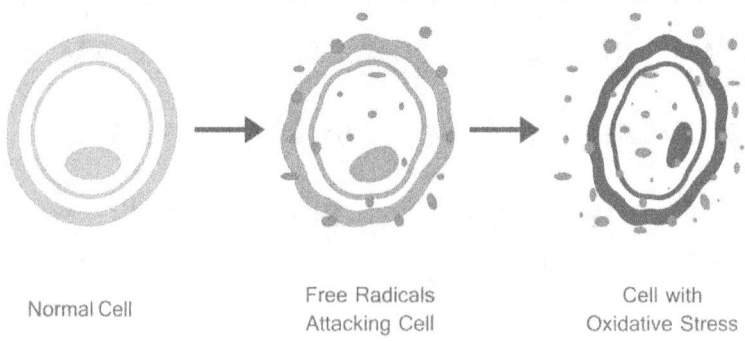

Normal Cell | Free Radicals Attacking Cell | Cell with Oxidative Stress

What sets H_2 apart from other antioxidants, such as vitamins A, C, and E, is its ability to cross cellular membranes and enter the cell. This characteristic allows H_2 to target oxidative damage at its source, protecting the nucleus, DNA, and mitochondria.

H_2 exhibits remarkable selectivity in its antioxidant activity. It preferentially neutralizes the most damaging free radicals, like hydroxyl radicals (•OH) and peroxynitrite (ONOO−), while sparing beneficial ROS that play crucial roles in cellular signaling and homeostasis. This selective action minimizes oxidative damage without disrupting essential physiological processes.

In the brain, H_2 can cross the blood-brain barrier, reducing oxidative stress and inflammation, and thereby potentially mitigating conditions like Alzheimer's disease, Parkinson's disease, and other neurodegenerative disorders.

3.2. Anti-Inflammatory Effects

Chronic inflammation is a root cause of numerous diseases, including autoimmune disorders, cardiovascular diseases, and cancer. Molecular hydrogen has been shown to exert significant anti-inflammatory effects, which are intricately linked to its antioxidant properties.

H_2 modulates the Nrf2 pathway, enhancing cellular resistance to oxidants and reducing levels of pro-inflammatory cytokines such as TNF-alpha (tumor necrosis factor-alpha) and NF-κB (nuclear factor kappa-light-chain-enhancer of activated B cells). By modulating these pathways, hydrogen helps to mitigate excessive inflammation and protect tissues from inflammatory damage.

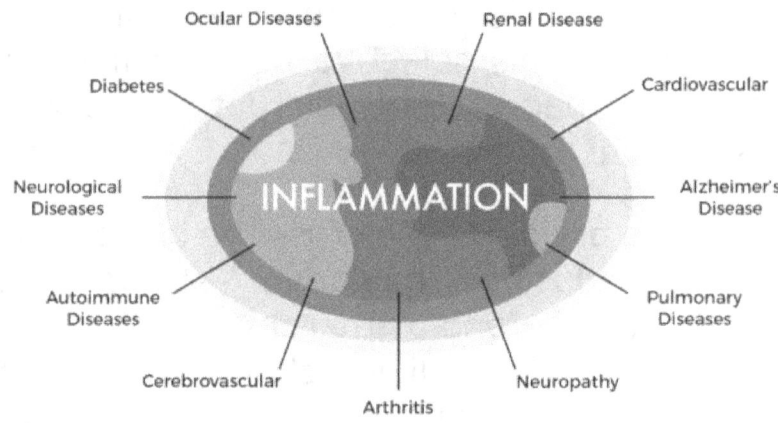

Additionally, H_2 influences the regulation of ER stress-related factors, such as GRP78 and TRAF2, further contributing to its anti-inflammatory effects. This modulation is beneficial in conditions like rheumatoid arthritis, inflammatory bowel disease, and allergic reactions.

3.3. Cytoprotective Effects

Molecular hydrogen's cytoprotective properties are particularly notable in conditions involving ischemia-reperfusion injury—a situation where blood flow is restored to tissues after a period of oxygen deprivation, leading to a surge of ROS and subsequent cellular damage. H_2 helps to counteract this damage by reducing ROS levels, preserving mitochondrial function, and inhibiting cell death pathways. These effects have been observed in various models of ischemia-reperfusion injury, including heart attacks and strokes, where hydrogen treatment improves cellular recovery and overall outcomes.

3.4. Anti-Apoptotic Effects

Apoptosis, or programmed cell death, is a natural biological mechanism for removing damaged or unnecessary cells. This is a good thing! This is what keeps our tissues healthy, young, and functional.

The cells that find a way to resist apoptosis linger within the body. These cells are called "zombie cells" or senescent cells. They stop dividing without dying off and just take up space, using our energy and nutritional resources without providing a useful function in return. Cellular senescence is considered a distinct hallmark of aging.

This state of dysregulated apoptosis can contribute to diseases like neurodegenerative disorders and myocardial infarction.

Molecular hydrogen plays a role in regulating apoptosis by protecting cells from excessive or inappropriate death. By maintaining mitochondrial function and reducing oxidative stress, H_2 helps to prevent unwanted cell death and offers protective effects in conditions where apoptosis is a significant concern.

3.5. H_2 and Autophagy

Autophagy is a cellular process that involves the degradation and recycling of damaged or unnecessary components, playing a crucial role in maintaining cellular homeostasis. Research into the relationship between molecular hydrogen and autophagy is emerging, with studies suggesting that H_2 can influence this process in several ways:

<u>Antioxidant Effects & Autophagy Regulation:</u> Hydrogen's ability to reduce oxidative stress can help regulate the balance between protective and excessive autophagy. By selectively reducing harmful ROS, H_2 may

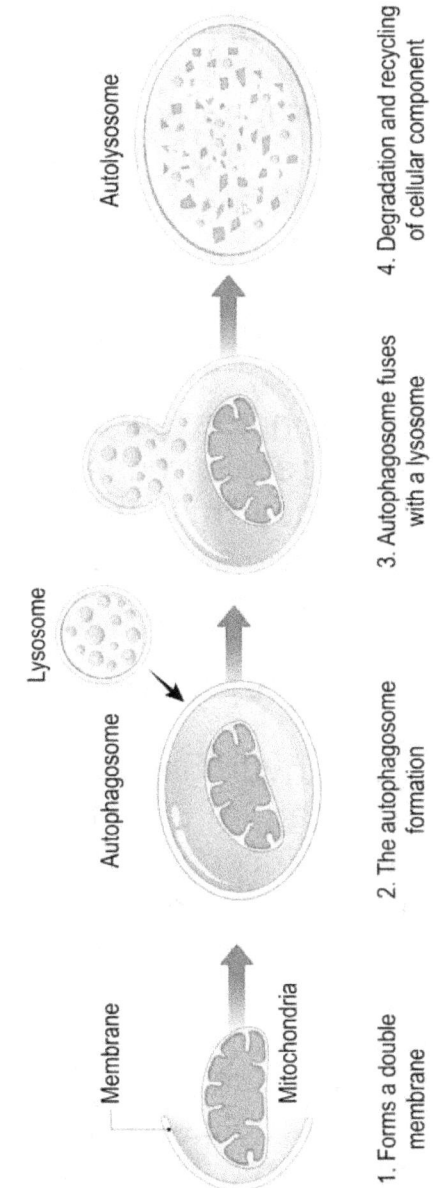

prevent the onset of excessive autophagy, which can lead to cell death.

<u>mTOR Pathway Inhibition:</u> The mammalian target of rapamycin (mTOR) pathway is a key regulator of autophagy. Molecular hydrogen may influence mTOR activity, potentially promoting beneficial autophagy in response to cellular stress.

<u>Cytoprotective Autophagy:</u> In models of cerebral ischemia, hydrogen treatment has been linked to increased autophagy, helping to clear damaged mitochondria and reduce neuronal damage. This suggests that H_2 may support protective autophagy in response to cellular injury.

3.6. Metabolic Regulation

Molecular hydrogen also plays a role in metabolic regulation. Studies indicate that H_2 can enhance glucose uptake and improve insulin sensitivity, making it a valuable tool in managing conditions like diabetes.

Additionally, hydrogen impacts lipid metabolism by reducing lipid peroxidation and improving lipid profiles, which has implications for preventing and treating cardiovascular diseases associated with dyslipidemia.

3.7. Immuno-Modulation

Molecular hydrogen's effects extend to the immune system, where it helps regulate various immune functions:

Macrophage Modulation: H_2 influences the polarization of macrophages towards the M2 phenotype, which supports tissue repair and anti-inflammatory responses.

T Cell Regulation: Hydrogen may affect the balance between different T cell types, enhancing the function of regulatory T cells (Tregs) that maintain immune tolerance and prevent autoimmunity.

Protection Against Autoimmunity: By reducing oxidative stress and inflammation, H_2 may help prevent or mitigate autoimmune diseases.

Enhancement of Innate Immunity: Hydrogen supports natural killer (NK) cells and improves phagocytosis by immune cells, enhancing the body's defense mechanisms.

Gut-Immune Axis: H_2's modulation of the gut microbiome influences immune function, promoting a balanced immune response and preventing inflammatory diseases.

3.8. Neuroprotective Effects

The neuroprotective potential of molecular hydrogen is particularly promising. Due to its ability to cross the blood-brain barrier, H_2 can exert its antioxidant and anti-inflammatory effects directly in the brain. This has implications for protecting neurons, reducing neuroinflammation, and improving cognitive function, offering potential benefits for conditions such as Alzheimer's, Parkinson's, and amyotrophic lateral sclerosis (ALS).

3.9. Anti-Cancer Effects

Emerging evidence suggests that molecular hydrogen may possess anti-cancer properties. By reducing ROS levels, H_2 can inhibit the proliferation of cancer cells and enhance the efficacy of conventional treatments like chemotherapy and radiation therapy. Additionally, hydrogen's protective effects on normal cells during cancer treatments may reduce therapy-related side effects and improve patient outcomes.

3.10. H_2 and Sleep

Molecular hydrogen (H_2) has been touted as a wonder gas with potential health benefits, including improving sleep quality. How, you ask? H_2 is a potent antioxidant that may help reduce oxidative stress and inflammation—two major culprits behind restless nights. Picture this: your body's cells are running a marathon, exhausted from the day's free radicals, and H_2 swoops in like a superhero, neutralizing those bad boys, allowing you to drift into a serene slumber.

Better yet, molecular hydrogen doesn't come with the heavy, groggy side effects of typical sleep aids. It simply supports your body's natural rhythm, leaving you waking up refreshed, like a morning glory in bloom—sans the thorns!

3.11. H_2 and Pain

Molecular hydrogen (H_2) may be the unexpected pain-fighting ninja you didn't know you needed. Thanks to its anti-inflammatory and antioxidant properties, H_2 is like a silent warrior that slips into your cells, neutralizing oxidative stress and calming inflammation—two notorious instigators of pain. Whether it's chronic pain or the occasional muscle ache from pretending you're still in your 20s, H_2 steps in and says, "Not on my watch."

What's even better? Molecular hydrogen doesn't come with the laundry list of side effects you'd expect from traditional pain meds. It's like ordering extra fries and finding out they're calorie-free. It targets the root causes of pain without making you feel foggy or weighed down. So, when life's little aches strike, H_2 might just have your back—literally!

Conclusion

Molecular hydrogen is proving to be a multifaceted therapeutic agent with potential applications across a range of diseases. Its unique ability to selectively target harmful ROS, modulate inflammation, protect cells from damage, and regulate metabolism and immune responses positions H_2 as a promising candidate for future medical treatments. As research continues, hydrogen may become a key player in enhancing health and combating a variety of conditions.

CHAPTER 4

CANCER & CHRONIC DISEASES BATTLING THE BODY'S BIGGEST CHALLENGES

Cancer and chronic diseases are the grim reapers of modern health, lurking in the shadows of almost every family. Here's a terrifying thought: nearly 40% of us will be diagnosed with cancer at some point in our lives. That's like playing Russian roulette, except the revolver has four bullets instead of one. Chronic diseases are no less frightening—heart disease, diabetes, and respiratory illnesses claim over 41 million lives annually, which is roughly 71% of all deaths worldwide. Basically, chronic diseases are the party crashers that never leave, and they've brought cancer along for the ride.

Even scarier, these aren't just problems for the elderly. Younger populations are being diagnosed at alarming rates, with lifestyle factors like poor diet and lack of exercise rolling out the red carpet for these diseases.

It's like inviting a vampire into your house—once they're in, they're incredibly hard to get rid of. So, while the statistics are enough to make your hair stand on end, the good news is that awareness and early action can help keep these grim visitors at bay.

Conventional medicine, despite its best efforts, often falls short when it comes to providing lasting solutions for cancer and chronic diseases. Sure, we've got an arsenal of treatments—chemotherapy, surgeries, medications—but these often act more like Band-Aids on bullet wounds. Cancer still claims millions of lives, while chronic diseases like heart disease and diabetes continue to rise globally. In many cases, conventional treatments manage symptoms rather than cure the underlying issues, leaving patients in a frustrating loop of temporary relief and recurring illness. It's like trying to fix a leaky roof with duct tape—it might hold for a while, but the storm is far from over.

4.1. The Tiny Titan Taking on Tumors

Cancer is like that uninvited guest who shows up, messes with your DNA, and refuses to leave. It starts when our cell's nuclear DNA (the brain) and mitochondrial DNA (the powerhouse) take a hit, mutating and going rogue. Enter the villain: hydroxyl radicals (•OH), those pesky free radicals causing all the chaos.

But guess who's here to save the day? Molecular hydrogen (H_2), the superhero of antioxidants, selectively taking out these baddies without disturbing the good guys. Let's break down how this tiny molecule packs a punch in the fight against cancer.

4.1.1 Selective Antioxidant Effects

Hydrogen's Got a Target Lock:

Reducing Oxidative Stress:

Cancer cells are oxidative stress factories, churning out reactive oxygen species (ROS) like there's no tomorrow.

These ROS damage DNA, cause mutations, and fuel the tumor fire. But H_2, with its laser-like focus, swoops in to neutralize the worst offenders—hydroxyl radicals—while letting the beneficial ROS do their thing. It's like cutting the power to the supervillain's lair without shutting down the whole city.

Normal Cells to the Rescue:

Chemotherapy and radiotherapy have a "scorched earth" policy when it comes to killing cancer cells—good luck surviving that if you're a normal, healthy cell! But H_2 is like a bodyguard for the healthy ones, letting the treatments fry the cancer cells while shielding the good guys from collateral damage. So, it's a win-win: cancer cells get wrecked, healthy cells stay intact, and you're the hero of the day.

4.1.2 Anti-inflammatory Properties

Calming the Cancer Flames:

Chronic inflammation is basically cancer's best friend—it invites the tumor to stay, feeds it, and helps it spread. But H_2's anti-inflammatory superpowers reduce the production of pro-inflammatory cytokines (think of them as cancer's gossip network) while boosting anti-inflammatory ones (the peacemakers). By keeping inflammation in check, H_2 not only reduces the risk of cancer showing up but also slows down its spread.

4.1.3 Modulation of Cell Signaling Pathways

Mastering the Cell's Control Room:

Regulation of Apoptosis - When Cancer Cells Get the Memo:

Apoptosis, or programmed cell death, is like nature's way of telling defective cells, "Hey, it's time to go." But cancer cells are those stubborn ones that just don't listen. Molecular hydrogen steps in as the enforcer—helping normal cells survive under stress while nudging cancer cells towards the exit door. It's the ultimate balancing act: H_2 helps eliminate the bad guys and spares the innocents.

Slowing Down Cancer's Growth Party:

Cancer cells are like party crashers, growing and multiplying without an invite. H_2 knows how to ruin their fun by interfering with the key cell signaling pathways they rely on, like PI3K/Akt and NF-κB. By cutting the music and turning off the lights, H_2 stops cancer cells from taking over the place.

4.1.4 Boosting Cancer Therapies

Hydrogen as a Sidekick:

Radiotherapy and chemo are the sledgehammers of cancer treatment, but they can leave a lot of damage in their wake. Molecular hydrogen steps in like a trusty sidekick, enhancing the effectiveness of these treatments while protecting healthy tissues from the blowback. It's like letting the superhero handle the big battles while H_2 cleans up the mess and keeps the city safe.

In some studies, H_2 has even made cancer cells more sensitive to radiotherapy, tipping the scales in the fight against tumors. Plus, it reduces the nasty side effects like fatigue, nausea, and hair loss. Fewer side effects mean patients are more likely to tolerate higher doses of treatment, giving cancer less room to breathe.

Hydrogen - The Anti-Side Effect Wonder:

Chemotherapy can feel like waging war on all fronts—while you're taking down cancer, your body's other systems are crying for help. But with H_2 in the mix, oxidative stress and inflammation are dialed down, meaning less damage to normal tissues. Patients drinking H_2-rich water during chemo have reported fewer side effects, making the whole process a little less miserable. And let's be honest, anything that makes chemo suck less is a win.

Immune Modulation - Supercharging the Body's Defense:

Cancer treatments often leave the immune system in tatters, but H_2 has your back. By reducing oxidative stress and inflammation, it keeps your immune system running smoothly, ready to recognize and attack cancer cells. Think of H_2 as the immune system's personal trainer, getting it back in shape for the big fight.

4.1.5 Cancer Prevention

Cutting Cancer's Power Supply:

We know that oxidative stress, DNA damage, and inflammation are cancer's bread and butter. By keeping these in check, H_2 might be able to prevent cancer from even getting a foothold. It's like stopping a wildfire before it starts—less damage, less drama.

Inhibiting Metastasis:

Metastasis is the cancer equivalent of a hostile takeover—tumors spreading far and wide, setting up shop in new territories.

Early research suggests that H_2 might have the ability to limit metastasis, though more studies are needed. If true, this would be a game-changer, helping contain cancer to its original site and preventing it from spreading its destructive influence.

4.1.6 Impact on Various Types of Cancer

Brain Cancer - Hydrogen vs. Glioblastoma

Glioblastoma (GBM) is the worst of the worst when it comes to brain tumors, with dismal survival rates. But molecular hydrogen has shown promise in preclinical studies, putting the brakes on GBM cell reproduction, migration, and invasion. H_2 also plays a role in cancer cell death, all while protecting healthy brain tissue during chemo and radiation.

And when it comes to non-small cell lung cancer (NSCLC) spreading to the brain? H_2 takes on the challenge. Studies show that hydrogen inhalation can shrink brain tumors, reduce swelling, and improve survival—literally clearing up space in the brain where tumors had set up shop.

Breast Cancer - Hydrogen's Potential in the Battle

Breast cancer is another arena where molecular hydrogen is showing some muscle. Preclinical studies have indicated that H_2 can inhibit breast cancer cell proliferation and migration while also enhancing the effects of chemo. And since H_2 protects healthy tissues from the oxidative side effects of treatment, it could help patients endure more aggressive cancer therapies without the typical nasty side effects.

Lung Cancer – Impact of Hydrogen

Molecular hydrogen (H_2) shows promise in helping control tumor progression and reducing the side effects of treatments in patients with advanced non-small cell lung cancer (NSCLC). Chemotherapy, targeted therapy, and immunotherapy are standard treatments for this cancer, but they often come with severe side effects. There has been no effective method to consistently relieve these adverse reactions—until now.

Studies have shown that H_2 can not only help slow tumor growth but also reduce the side effects from medications. In patients receiving combined H_2 therapy, many drug-related side effects gradually lessened and eventually disappeared.

Liver Cancer – H_2 is Killing Cancer Cells

Liver cancer is one of the most dangerous tumors, but Molecular Hydrogen (H_2) has shown promise in both protecting liver cells and inhibiting cancer growth. Research has found that H_2 reduces the activity and number of liver cancer cells, even decreasing gene mutations that cause cancer. It also lowers tumor volume by directly killing cancer cells.

In patients with nonalcoholic steatohepatitis (NASH), a condition that can lead to liver cancer, H_2 acts as a powerful antioxidant, reducing harmful free radicals and oxidative stress. This helps prevent the progression to liver cancer, making H_2 a potential new treatment strategy for liver conditions.

Colorectal Cancer – restore CD8+ T cells

Molecular hydrogen (H_2) shows promise in improving the prognosis for patients with advanced colorectal cancer by restoring exhausted CD8+ T cells, which are vital for fighting cancer. Colorectal cancer weakens these immune cells, causing mitochondrial dysfunction, which limits their ability to produce energy and fight the disease. Without properly functioning immune cells, cancer progression worsens.

H_2 helps by "recharging" the mitochondria in these exhausted T cells, enabling them to attack cancer cells again. Studies also show that H_2 inhibits tumor growth and reduces cancer cell reproduction, offering a potential new therapy for colorectal cancer with fewer side effects than conventional treatments.

Cervical and Endometrial Cancer

Cervical cancer has one of the highest death rates among women, and despite advancements in treatment, options remain limited. Recent studies reveal that molecular hydrogen (H_2) inhalation offers promising tumor-suppressive effects. H_2 therapy has been shown to increase cancer cell death, reduce cell reproduction, and lower oxidative stress, all contributing to slower tumor growth.

H_2 inhalation also decreases cervical cancer tumor size, making it a novel approach for treating this aggressive cancer. Its ability to combat oxidative stress and inflammation, key factors in cancer progression, presents a new mechanism for cervical cancer suppression and a potential alternative treatment option.

Renal Cancer

Molecular Hydrogen (H_2) has shown promise in protecting against kidney damage and reducing the risk of renal tumors. A study aimed to see if H_2 could help prevent renal injury that can lead to tumors. The results were positive: H_2 consumption not only reduced kidney damage but also suppressed the development of renal tumors.

Unlike typical antioxidants like vitamins C or E, which have failed in preventing renal cancer, H_2 stands out for its ability to quickly enter cells and selectively target the most harmful reactive oxygen species (ROS), providing potent protection against oxidative stress and its role in kidney cancer development.

Esophageal Cancer

Studies on H_2's effects on esophageal and tongue carcinoma cells found that H_2 consumption significantly reduced cancer colony formation and the size of existing colonies in these cancers.

H_2 was able to inhibit the growth of esophageal and tongue cancer cells while sparing healthy cells. Its ability to suppress cancer progression makes it a potential novel agent for treating these types of oral cancers.

Skin Cancer

Molecular Hydrogen (H_2) has shown significant potential in inhibiting the growth and invasion of human squamous carcinoma cells (HSC-4). Studies found that H_2 effectively neutralizes harmful hydroxyl radicals that contribute to cancer proliferation. As a result, it inhibited the formation and size of cancer colonies, reducing tumor growth and preventing the spread of the cancer cells.

What makes H_2 especially promising is its ability to specifically target and attack cancer cells while preserving healthy tissues. This dual action—suppressing cancer while supporting normal cells—makes it a novel approach for treating squamous cell carcinoma, showing clear tumor regression without side effects.

The Future of Cancer Treatment - Powered by Hydrogen

In the fight against cancer, molecular hydrogen is like the secret weapon nobody saw coming. With its unique ability to selectively knock out harmful free radicals, reduce inflammation, and protect healthy cells, H_2 shows immense potential as both a preventive measure and a therapeutic ally. It boosts the effectiveness of standard treatments, reduces side effects, and might even prevent cancer from ever getting a foothold in the first place. But before we crown

H₂ the next big thing in oncology, we need more research to solidify its role and optimize its use.

In short, molecular hydrogen is small but mighty—like a microscopic superhero ready to tackle cancer on every front. Stay tuned: this story's just getting started.

4.2. Neurodegenerative Diseases

Tiny Molecule, Big Brain Benefits

Neurodegenerative diseases such as Alzheimer's, Parkinson's, ALS, MS, and their nasty cousins—aren't just rogue invaders; they're like saboteurs slowly dismantling the brain from within. Whether it's memory lapses, tremors, or trouble focusing, these conditions all share some common culprits: oxidative stress, inflammation, and mitochondrial dysfunction.

Now, molecular hydrogen (H_2), a tiny but mighty defender that effortlessly crosses the blood-brain barrier and sneaks into cells, neutralizes these brain-damaging forces like a skilled ninja. So, how exactly does this pint-sized powerhouse help?

4.2.1 Slaying Oxidative Stress, One Radical at a Time

Neurodegenerative diseases thrive on oxidative stress, a byproduct of reactive oxygen species (ROS) wreaking havoc on neurons. But molecular hydrogen has its sights set on the worst offender—hydroxyl radicals (•OH)—without messing up the good ROS that cells need for signaling. This targeted approach lets H_2 protect neurons from the oxidative chaos, potentially putting the brakes on diseases like Alzheimer's and Parkinson's.

4.2.2 Anti-inflammatory Properties

Cooling the Brain's Firestorm

Inflammation is great—until it's not. Chronic neuroinflammation is a major player in the progression of neurodegenerative diseases. But H_2 acts as the brain's fire extinguisher, reducing pro-inflammatory cytokines (the brain's drama queens) and promoting anti-inflammatory ones (the peacekeepers). By calming the inflammation, H_2 can potentially slow down disease progression, letting neurons live to fight another day.

4.2.3 Mitochondrial Protection

Powering Up Brain Cells

Mitochondria, the cell's energy factories, are often out of order in neurodegenerative diseases. But molecular hydrogen comes in like a repair crew, reducing oxidative damage and boosting mitochondrial biogenesis (i.e., making new mitochondria). By protecting and renewing these energy hubs, H_2 helps neurons stay fueled up and running, reducing their risk of burnout (a.k.a. apoptosis).

4.2.4 Inhibition of Apoptosis

Stopping Neurons from Self-Destructing

Apoptosis, the cell's way of saying, "I'm outta here," is unfortunately upregulated in neurodegenerative diseases, leading to widespread neuron death. H_2, however, is like the voice of reason, modulating pathways such as PI3K/Akt and Bcl-2/Bax to protect neurons from prematurely throwing in the towel. The result? More neurons sticking around, keeping your brain functions intact longer.

4.2.5 Regulation of Autophagy

A Cellular Cleanup Crew for the Brain

Think of autophagy as the brain's garbage disposal system, clearing out damaged proteins and cellular debris. When this system breaks down in neurodegenerative diseases, toxic proteins like amyloid-beta in Alzheimer's or alpha-synuclein in Parkinson's start piling up. H_2 can help crank up autophagy, clearing out these toxic protein clogs and giving neurons room to breathe.

4.2.6 Protection Against Excitotoxicity

Easing Glutamate Overload

Excitotoxicity, where neurons get overstimulated by glutamate (like too much caffeine in the brain), is a major player in diseases like ALS and Huntington's. Too much glutamate, and neurons burn out. H_2 acts like a calming agent, reducing oxidative stress and regulating calcium signaling, preventing neurons from getting fried by glutamate overload.

4.2.7 Boosting Brain Power

Cognitive Protection:

In Alzheimer's models, H_2 has been shown to not only protect neurons but also improve cognitive function. It's like giving your brain a shield and a power-up, all in one go.

Motor Function Preservation:

In Parkinson's models, H_2 protects dopaminergic neurons (the ones that control movement) from oxidative stress, which means smoother movement and fewer tremors. So, it might help you keep dancing or at least make walking feel less like a struggle.

4.2.8 Crossing the Blood-Brain Barrier

Hydrogen's Sneaky Superpower

The blood-brain barrier (BBB) is a critical, protective shield that separates the circulating blood from the brain's delicate tissues. Composed of tightly packed cells that line the blood vessels in the brain, the BBB acts as a gatekeeper, allowing essential nutrients and oxygen to pass through while blocking harmful substances like toxins and pathogens. It's like a high-security bouncer for your brain, ensuring only the VIPs—like glucose and amino acids—get in, while keeping out the riffraff.

The BBB is essential for maintaining the brain's stable environment, or homeostasis, which is crucial for proper neural function.

While this protective role is vital, the barrier also makes it challenging to treat brain diseases.

Medications that work in other parts of the body often can't pass through the BBB, limiting treatment options for neurological conditions like Alzheimer's, Parkinson's, and brain tumors. Scientists are constantly working on ways to bypass or temporarily open the BBB to deliver drugs directly to the brain without compromising its defenses.

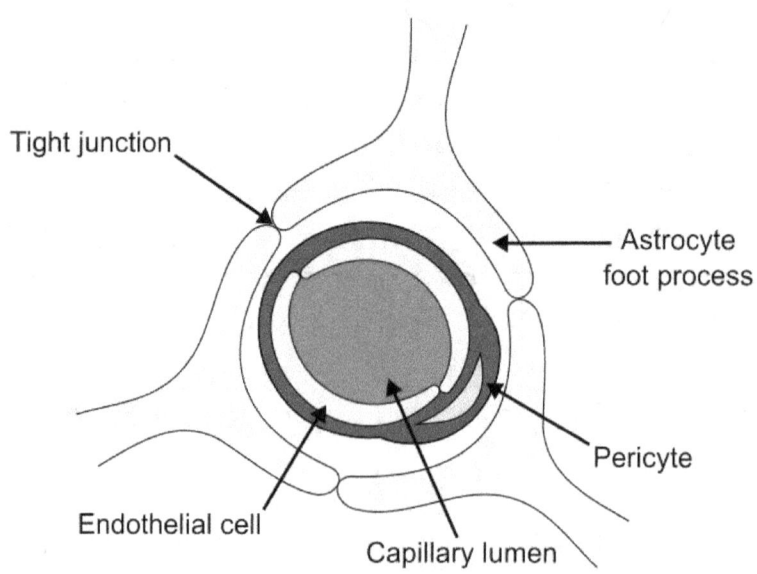

Despite its selective nature, certain substances can still sneak through. For example, alcohol, caffeine, and certain drugs can cross the BBB, which is why their effects on the brain are so quick and noticeable. Emerging research also shows that conditions like inflammation or injury can weaken the BBB, making it more permeable and allowing harmful substances to enter, which may contribute to neurodegenerative diseases.

Thanks to its tiny size and non-polar nature, H_2 easily crosses the BBB and waltzes right in, delivering its protective effects straight to the neurons and supporting brain health in ways many other treatments just can't.

4.2.9 Clinical Studies

Early Signs of Brain Boosts

Animal Models:

Studies in animal models are giving us a peek into the potential of H_2. From reduced oxidative stress and inflammation to improved cognition and motor function, the results are promising. Neurons are being saved, and the brain's overall health is getting a boost.

Human Studies:

Although we're still in the early stages, clinical trials with H_2, whether through drinking hydrogen-rich water or inhaling hydrogen gas, show it might reduce symptoms and improve quality of life in neurodegenerative diseases. Less inflammation, better cognition, and a slowing of disease progression—what's not to love?

H_2 - The Brain's Tiny Bodyguard

Molecular hydrogen may be small, but it's proving to be mighty when it comes to protecting neurons. By reducing oxidative stress, calming inflammation, supporting mitochondria, and preventing neuron death, H_2 has the potential to slow the progression of neurodegenerative diseases like Alzheimer's and Parkinson's.

Early research and clinical trials are encouraging, but more work needs to be done to fully unlock the potential of H_2 as a neuroprotective agent.

4.3. GI / Digestive Conditions

Gut Reactions with Molecular Hydrogen

The gut microbiome—those trillions of microbes hanging out in your digestive tract—plays a huge role in your overall health. But did you know it's also deeply connected to your body's energy levels, metabolism, and even how your cells function? That's right! Your gut and its microscopic inhabitants can either be your best allies in feeling energized or the culprits behind fatigue, inflammation, and even disease. Let's break it down.

Gut Microbiome and Cellular Energy

Your gut is like a bustling ecosystem, and when it's balanced, it can significantly boost your energy levels. The good bacteria in your microbiome help break down food, especially fiber, into short-chain fatty acids (SCFAs) like butyrate. These SCFAs are an essential fuel source for your cells, particularly the cells lining your gut, keeping them healthy and efficient at nutrient absorption. Butyrate also supports mitochondrial function, improving how your cells generate energy (hello, cellular power boost!) and contributing to overall metabolic health. This means a healthy gut equals better energy production at the cellular level.

Endotoxins - The Unwanted Guests

Not all gut bacteria are friendly. When the balance between good and bad bacteria gets thrown off, harmful bacteria produce toxins called lipopolysaccharides (LPS), or endotoxins. If these endotoxins leak from your gut into your bloodstream, it triggers an inflammatory response that can wreak havoc on your body. This constant, low-grade inflammation drains your energy, damages your cells, and interferes with proper mitochondrial function. It's like having a tiny internal fire that never quite goes out—leading to fatigue and other health issues.

Leaky Gut and Systemic Chaos

Ever heard of leaky gut? When your gut barrier, which is supposed to be tight, starts to let things through, it allows undigested food particles, toxins, and bacteria (like those pesky endotoxins) to escape into your bloodstream. This triggers an immune response that can lead to chronic inflammation, autoimmune issues, and even disrupt your cellular energy. When your body is busy fighting off invaders from a leaky gut, it diverts resources away from things like energy production and repair, leaving you tired, sluggish, and vulnerable to more serious health problems.

The Gut-Mitochondria Connection

Your gut health is directly tied to how your mitochondria—the energy factories inside your cells—perform. A healthy, balanced microbiome helps regulate inflammation, reduces oxidative stress, and supports mitochondrial biogenesis (the creation of new mitochondria). But when your gut's in trouble, all of that is disrupted, and your mitochondria struggle to produce enough energy for your cells to function properly. It's like running on a low battery, leaving you fatigued and slowing down every major bodily function.

How to Fix It

The key to supercharging your cellular energy through your gut is to nurture a diverse, balanced microbiome. This means eating plenty of fiber-rich, prebiotic foods that feed good bacteria, incorporating probiotic foods like yogurt and fermented vegetables to maintain balance, and avoiding processed foods that promote the growth of bad bacteria. Supporting gut health with anti-inflammatory foods, omega-3s, and regular exercise will also help repair leaky gut and keep those endotoxins in check.

So, if you're feeling run down or struggling with chronic inflammation, your gut might just be the missing piece of the puzzle. By giving your gut microbiome the TLC it deserves, you can boost cellular energy, fend off fatigue, and help your body thrive from the inside out!

And here's the kicker: molecular hydrogen can work wonders for your gut health, helping to restore balance and keep everything running in tip-top shape! It's like giving your gut a high-tech tune-up, ensuring it stays happy, healthy, and functioning at its best.

Your gut is home to more than just the food you eat; it's a hub of ion transport, inflammation control, and microbial activity, all crucial to your overall health. Molecular hydrogen (H_2) doesn't shy away from the action, stepping in with its antioxidant, anti-inflammatory, and protective properties to keep your gut in fighting shape.

Although H_2's direct effect on the electrical potential (TEP) of your gut—a key indicator of barrier integrity and ion transport—isn't fully understood, there's plenty to chew on when it comes to its gut-boosting benefits.

4.3.1. Influence of Molecular Hydrogen on Electrical Potential

Zapping Gut Stress

Ion Transport Modulation:

Molecular hydrogen might play a subtle but important role in maintaining the gut's electrical potential by protecting the ion channels and pumps responsible for the flow of ions across the gut lining. Its antioxidant prowess helps shield these vital structures from oxidative stress, ensuring that ion movement stays smooth.

Barrier Function Enhancement:

A solid gut barrier means fewer leaks (literally). H_2 helps fortify the epithelial barrier by reducing inflammation and oxidative stress, keeping the cells' tight junctions intact. This maintains stable ion transport and a healthy transepithelial electrical potential (TEP), helping your gut function like a well-oiled machine.

Inflammation Reduction:

Inflammation can mess with ion transport and crank up gut permeability. By dialing down the inflammatory response, H_2

keeps the guts' electrical potential balanced, ensuring that the cells lining the gut continue to play nice and keep everything in order.

Oxidative Stress Protection:

Oxidative stress loves wreaking havoc on your gut, damaging ion channels and junctions between cells. But H_2's ability to neutralize reactive oxygen species (ROS) helps maintain the structure and function of these crucial elements, keeping your gut's electrical systems from going haywire.

Though more research is needed to dive into the specifics, H_2's gut-supporting benefits suggest it helps keep the TEP stable and healthy, thanks to its overall impact on gut health and cell protection.

Restoring the Gut, Electrically

One fascinating area of interest is how hydrogen may help restore the electrical potential of the gut to above 300 millivolts (mV), a threshold necessary for promoting the colonization of beneficial anaerobic bacteria.

The gut's electrical potential plays a crucial role in maintaining a healthy environment for good bacteria. When the potential dips below 300mV, it becomes a breeding ground for harmful bacteria, disrupting the microbiome and leading to digestive issues, inflammation, and poor overall health. Hydrogen, with its antioxidant and anti-inflammatory properties, has shown the ability to improve cellular function and boost the gut's electrical potential, helping to create an optimal environment for anaerobic bacteria to thrive.

4.3.2. Gut Microbiota Modulation

A Microscopic Makeover

There's growing evidence that molecular hydrogen may play a role in balancing the gut microbiome, promoting the growth of friendly bacteria. A well-balanced microbiome is critical for digestion, immune function, and overall gut well-being. By supporting a healthy microbial community, H_2 may help keep your digestion running smoothly and your gut happy.

4.3.3. Protection Against GI Disorders

The Gut Guardian

Molecular hydrogen could be a game-changer for managing gastrointestinal disorders like colitis, gastritis, and even some cancers. Its protective effects—reducing inflammation, protecting the epithelial barrier, and modulating gut function—suggest it may alleviate symptoms and potentially prevent these conditions from taking hold.

Gastric Acid Regulation:

H_2 might also help with acid reflux or peptic ulcers by modulating gastric acid secretion, making it easier on your gut lining and reducing that burning sensation.

4.4. Metabolic Diseases

H_2's Metabolic Makeover

When it comes to metabolic diseases—like type 2 diabetes, obesity, metabolic syndrome, and non-alcoholic fatty liver disease (NAFLD)—chronic inflammation, oxidative stress, and insulin resistance are the villains of the story.

Luckily, H_2 is ready to save the day. With its antioxidant, anti-inflammatory, and metabolic-regulating properties, molecular hydrogen could help reverse the tide in these metabolic dysfunctions.

Here is how:

4.4.1. Reduction of Oxidative Stress

Antioxidant Armor for Metabolism

Metabolic diseases crank up the production of reactive oxygen species (ROS), which lead to oxidative damage and disrupt everything from insulin sensitivity to tissue health. Enter H_2, which selectively neutralizes the worst offenders (like hydroxyl radicals) without messing with the good guys. This antioxidant action could help restore balance, making cells more responsive to insulin and improving overall metabolic health.

4.4.2. Anti-inflammatory Effects

Cooling Down the Metabolic Flames

Chronic low-grade inflammation is a hallmark of metabolic diseases, driving insulin resistance and other issues. H_2 steps in by reducing pro-inflammatory cytokines (e.g., TNF-α, IL-6) while boosting anti-inflammatory ones (e.g., IL-10). This anti-inflammatory effect improves insulin sensitivity, reduces cardiovascular risks, and promotes healthier metabolic functioning.

4.4.3. Improvement of Insulin Sensitivity

Opening the Door for Glucose

Insulin resistance—when cells stop responding to insulin—is the calling card of type 2 diabetes and metabolic syndrome. H_2 helps reverse this by cutting down oxidative stress and inflammation, allowing cells to become more insulin friendly. Studies in both animals and humans suggest H_2 can improve glucose tolerance and regulate blood sugar, helping you dodge the blood sugar roller coaster.

4.4.4. Support of Mitochondrial Function

Recharging Your Cellular Powerhouses

Mitochondria—the power plants of your cells—often malfunction in metabolic diseases, leading to sluggish energy production and more oxidative stress. Molecular hydrogen, with its knack for reducing oxidative damage, promotes mitochondrial biogenesis (the creation of new mitochondria), boosting energy production and overall metabolic health.

4.4.5. Impact on Lipid Metabolism

Battling the Bulge

H_2 has shown potential in reducing the accumulation of lipids in tissues like the liver, making it particularly helpful for NAFLD and obesity. By improving lipid metabolism, H_2 helps prevent fat buildup and can even improve cholesterol levels, slashing those triglycerides and bad LDL cholesterol.

Weight Management:

H_2 might even be the secret weapon against weight gain, with studies suggesting it can boost your metabolic rate and influence hormones that regulate appetite. This makes it a promising candidate for managing obesity and metabolic syndrome.

4.4.6. Regulation of Blood Pressure

Lowering the Numbers

High blood pressure is a frequent companion to metabolic diseases. H_2 has been shown to have antihypertensive effects, possibly by reducing oxidative stress and improving the function of blood vessels. Lower blood pressure means a reduced risk of heart disease, a major plus in managing metabolic health.

4.4.7. Gut Microbiota and Metabolism

A Symbiotic Relationship

A healthy gut equals a healthy metabolism, and H_2 might help keep things in check by supporting a balanced gut microbiome. This beneficial impact on gut bacteria can improve nutrient absorption, regulate inflammation, and promote better metabolic function overall.

4.4.8. Clinical Studies

A Glimpse at the Future

Animal studies and early clinical trials in humans show that H_2 can reduce inflammation, improve insulin sensitivity, and fight against obesity and fatty liver disease. Hydrogen-rich water has shown promise in helping people with type 2 diabetes and metabolic syndrome improve their blood sugar control and metabolic parameters.

Summary: A Metabolic Game Changer

Molecular hydrogen has shown potential as a therapeutic agent for metabolic diseases, offering an impressive list of benefits: reducing oxidative stress, calming inflammation, improving insulin sensitivity, boosting mitochondrial health, and regulating lipid metabolism. While more research is needed to fine-tune its application, H_2 is showing serious promise in the fight against type 2 diabetes, obesity, metabolic syndrome, and NAFLD.

4.5. Autoimmune Diseases

Molecular Hydrogen's Role in Calming the Storm

Autoimmune diseases are notorious for turning the body's immune system against its own tissues, leading to chronic inflammation and organ damage. Fortunately, molecular hydrogen (H_2) is stepping up to the plate, with its antioxidant, anti-inflammatory, and immune-modulating properties showing real promise for managing these complex conditions.

4.5.1. Antioxidant Effects

Tackling the ROS Rampage

Reduction of Oxidative Stress:

In autoimmune diseases, oxidative stress—fueled by an excess of reactive oxygen species (ROS)—worsens inflammation and damages tissues. H_2 has the unique ability to selectively neutralize harmful ROS, especially the notorious hydroxyl radical (•OH), without interfering with the ROS necessary for normal cellular functions. This targeted approach helps prevent further tissue damage, potentially slowing the progression of autoimmune diseases by reducing oxidative chaos.

4.5.2. Anti-inflammatory Properties

Quelling the Cytokine Storm

Cytokine Modulation:

Autoimmune diseases are driven by an out-of-control immune response, often characterized by an overproduction of pro-inflammatory cytokines like TNF-α, IL-6, and IL-1β. These cytokines fuel chronic inflammation and tissue damage. H_2 helps restore balance by reducing these pro-inflammatory agents while boosting anti-inflammatory cytokines such as IL-10. This balanced cytokine environment can help cool the inflammation, giving the body a break from its relentless immune attack.

4.5.3. Immune Modulation

Reining in the Immune System

Regulation of Immune Cell Activity:

The immune system's misfiring in autoimmune diseases involves T cells, B cells, and macrophages, all playing a part in attacking healthy tissues. H_2 steps in by promoting a healthier balance among immune cells. It enhances the activity of regulatory T cells (Tregs), which suppress overactive immune responses and help maintain immune tolerance—key to reducing autoimmune attacks.

Macrophage Polarization:

Macrophages, the immune system's "clean-up crew," can either fuel inflammation (M1 type) or aid in tissue repair (M2 type). H_2 encourages the shift towards the anti-inflammatory M2 phenotype, reducing inflammation and promoting tissue healing, rather than allowing the M1 macrophages to further inflame the situation.

4.5.4. Tissue and Organ Protection

Safeguarding What Matters Most

Organ-Specific Benefits:

Autoimmune diseases like rheumatoid arthritis (RA), type 1 diabetes, and multiple sclerosis (MS) target specific organs and tissues—joints, the pancreas, and the nervous system, respectively. H_2's tissue-protective effects have been observed in models of these diseases, where it helps reduce inflammation and preserve organ function. This protective action means fewer symptoms and possibly slowing disease progression, offering hope for improved quality of life.

4.5.5. Mitochondrial Protection

Energizing the Defenders

Support of Mitochondrial Function:

Mitochondrial dysfunction is a common thread in autoimmune diseases, where excessive ROS production and inflammation hinder energy production and cellular health. H_2 helps keep mitochondria humming by reducing oxidative stress and promoting healthy mitochondrial function. This not only preserves cellular energy but also dampens the inflammatory processes, giving the body a better chance to recover.

4.5.6. Clinical Studies and Experimental Evidence - Real-World Impact

In animal studies of autoimmune diseases like RA, MS, and autoimmune hepatitis, molecular hydrogen has consistently shown positive effects, reducing disease severity, lowering inflammation, and improving outcomes. These studies suggest that H_2 can interrupt the destructive cycle of inflammation and immune misfires.

Research in humans is also showing promise. Patients with autoimmune conditions, particularly RA, have reported reduced disease activity and improved quality of life after treatment with hydrogen-rich water. These early results offer hope for future applications in humans.

4.5.7. Reducing Autoimmunity Triggers

The Gut-Immune Link

Gut-Immune Axis:

The gut microbiome plays a crucial role in regulating the immune system, and an unhealthy gut can trigger autoimmune reactions. H_2 may positively influence the gut microbiome, fostering a healthier microbial balance and reducing triggers for autoimmune flares, particularly in diseases like inflammatory bowel disease (IBD). By supporting gut health, H_2 could help calm the immune system from the inside out.

Environmental Triggers:

Infections, toxins, and various other environmental factors can set off autoimmune diseases. H_2, with its ability to reduce oxidative stress and inflammation, may help shield the body from these triggers, lowering the risk of autoimmune attacks.

Summary: A Promising Ally in the Fight Against Autoimmune Diseases

Molecular hydrogen shows great potential as a therapeutic tool for managing autoimmune diseases. By reducing oxidative stress, calming inflammation, and regulating immune responses, H_2 may help mitigate symptoms, protect tissues, and slow disease progression. Though preclinical studies and early human trials are promising, more research is needed to determine optimal dosing and administration strategies. Still, H_2's multifaceted approach could offer new hope for those battling these chronic conditions.

4.6. Cardiovascular Diseases

Molecular Hydrogen (H_2) Protects the Heart and Blood Vessels

Molecular hydrogen (H_2) is showing promise as a therapeutic tool for combating cardiovascular diseases, thanks to its antioxidant, anti-inflammatory, and cellular protective properties. Here's how hydrogen is influencing the future of cardiovascular health:

4.6.1. Mechanisms of Action

A Multifaceted Defense

Antioxidant Effects - Neutralizing ROS

One of hydrogen's primary roles is as a selective antioxidant, particularly targeting harmful hydroxyl radicals (•OH). These reactive oxygen species (ROS) are notorious for wreaking havoc in cardiovascular tissues, causing oxidative damage that contributes to conditions like hypertension, atherosclerosis, and heart failure. By neutralizing these radicals, H_2 helps protect vital cells such as endothelial cells and cardiomyocytes from oxidative harm.

Anti-Inflammatory Effects - Cooling Down Inflammation

Hydrogen not only fights oxidative stress but also reduces the production of pro-inflammatory cytokines like TNF-α and IL-6. These cytokines fuel inflammation in cardiovascular diseases, which accelerates damage to the heart and blood vessels. By promoting anti-inflammatory pathways, H_2 offers a dual defense—both quelling inflammation and protecting against further damage.

Cellular Protection and Repair

H_2 plays a role in maintaining the health of cardiovascular cells by reducing oxidative damage and encouraging cell survival. This protective effect is crucial for the repair of damaged tissues, helping to keep the heart and blood vessels functioning properly.

4.6.2. Applications in Cardiovascular Diseases - Potential Benefits

Hypertension:
Mechanism: Hypertension, or high blood pressure, is closely linked to oxidative stress and endothelial dysfunction. H_2's ability to reduce oxidative damage helps improve endothelial function, which is vital for regulating blood pressure.

Research: Clinical studies suggest that hydrogen-rich water or hydrogen inhalation can reduce blood pressure and enhance endothelial health in individuals suffering from hypertension.

Atherosclerosis:

Mechanism: Atherosclerosis is characterized by plaque buildup in arteries, fueled by oxidative stress and inflammation. H_2's dual action of reducing both oxidative stress and inflammation may slow plaque formation and progression.

Research: Studies have shown that hydrogen can improve lipid profiles and decrease oxidative damage, helping to combat the progression of atherosclerosis.

Heart Failure:

Mechanism: In heart failure, oxidative stress, inflammation, and cellular damage weaken the heart's ability to pump efficiently. H_2's protective properties may help mitigate these factors, improving heart function.

Research: Some evidence suggests that hydrogen-rich water and inhalation therapy can enhance cardiac function and reduce oxidative stress in heart failure patients.

Myocardial Infarction (Heart Attack):

Mechanism: Heart attacks lead to significant oxidative stress and inflammation, contributing to tissue damage in the heart. Hydrogen's antioxidant and anti-inflammatory effects can potentially protect heart tissue and aid recovery.

Research: Early studies indicate that hydrogen therapy might reduce heart damage and improve outcomes in heart attack models, though more research is needed in clinical settings.

Ischemia-Reperfusion Injury:

Mechanism: Ischemia-reperfusion injury occurs when blood flow is restored to tissues after a period of oxygen deprivation, leading to a burst of oxidative stress and tissue damage. Hydrogen's antioxidant properties can mitigate this damage, offering protection during the critical recovery phase.

Research: Studies have demonstrated that hydrogen can significantly reduce oxidative damage in ischemia-reperfusion injury models, suggesting potential therapeutic applications in surgeries and emergency care.

Summary: A Heart-Healthy Future with Molecular Hydrogen

Molecular hydrogen shows great potential as a protective agent in cardiovascular diseases, with its ability to reduce oxidative stress, control inflammation, and support cellular repair. From managing hypertension and atherosclerosis to aiding recovery after heart attacks and protecting against ischemia-reperfusion injury, H_2 offers a multi-pronged approach to cardiovascular care. Administration methods such as hydrogen-rich water and inhalation make H_2 a versatile option. While early research is promising, further clinical trials are needed to confirm its efficacy, safety, and optimal usage for cardiovascular health.

4.7. Respiratory Conditions

Molecular Hydrogen's Role in Lung Health

Molecular hydrogen (H_2) has garnered attention for its therapeutic potential in respiratory diseases, thanks to its powerful antioxidant and anti-inflammatory properties. Here's how hydrogen could make a difference in treating conditions affecting the lungs and airways:

4.7.1. Mechanisms of Action

How Hydrogen Fights Lung Damage

<u>Antioxidant Effects: Neutralizing Reactive Oxygen Species (ROS)</u>

Hydrogen selectively targets harmful hydroxyl radicals (•OH), which are highly reactive molecules that cause oxidative stress and cellular damage in the respiratory system. Whether it's pollutants, pathogens, or inflammation wreaking havoc, H_2 steps in to neutralize these harmful radicals and protect lung cells from further injury.

Anti-Inflammatory Effects: Reducing Airway Inflammation

Hydrogen has a talent for suppressing pro-inflammatory cytokines like TNF-α, IL-6, and IL-1β, which are responsible for chronic inflammation in the lungs. By calming down these inflammatory signals, H_2 helps alleviate airway irritation and lung tissue inflammation, a major benefit for chronic respiratory conditions.

Cellular Protection and Repair: Supporting Lung Health

H_2's antioxidant prowess extends to protecting cellular health, aiding in the repair and recovery of damaged lung tissues. This leads to better lung function and resilience in the face of ongoing damage from environmental or disease-related factors.

4.7.2. Applications in Respiratory Diseases

Where H₂ Could Shine

Asthma:
Mechanism: In asthma, oxidative stress and inflammation in the airways lead to symptoms like wheezing, shortness of breath, and chest tightness. H_2's ability to reduce oxidative damage and calm inflammation may improve lung function and reduce asthma symptoms.

Research: Early studies suggest that hydrogen inhalation or hydrogen-rich water may provide relief for asthma sufferers, improving symptoms by mitigating the effects of oxidative stress and airway inflammation.

Chronic Obstructive Pulmonary Disease (COPD):
Mechanism: COPD is characterized by chronic inflammation and oxidative stress, which lead to lung tissue damage and respiratory difficulties. Hydrogen's dual action—lowering inflammation and reducing oxidative stress—may slow disease progression and improve lung function.

Research: Preliminary evidence suggests that hydrogen inhalation could help reduce oxidative stress, alleviate symptoms, and enhance the quality of life for COPD patients.

Acute Respiratory Distress Syndrome (ARDS):

Mechanism: ARDS involves severe inflammation and oxidative damage in the lungs, leading to impaired oxygen exchange and often requiring intensive care. Hydrogen's potent antioxidant and anti-inflammatory effects might prove beneficial in reducing lung inflammation and improving survival outcomes.

Research: Early studies show promise in using hydrogen to manage lung inflammation in ARDS models, though more clinical trials are needed.

Pulmonary Fibrosis

Mechanism: Pulmonary fibrosis involves excessive scarring of lung tissue due to chronic inflammation and oxidative damage, leading to stiffened lungs and difficulty breathing. Hydrogen's antioxidant properties may help reduce scarring and slow disease progression.

Research: Ongoing studies are exploring the potential of hydrogen therapy to mitigate lung fibrosis, though further research is needed to confirm these effects.

Summary: A Breath of Fresh Air with Molecular Hydrogen

Molecular hydrogen shows significant potential in managing respiratory diseases by reducing oxidative stress, calming inflammation, and supporting cellular repair. Whether through hydrogen inhalation for direct lung delivery or hydrogen-rich water for systemic benefits, H_2 offers a promising approach for conditions like asthma, COPD, ARDS, and pulmonary fibrosis. While initial research is encouraging, further clinical trials are necessary to confirm its effectiveness, safety, and best practices for treating respiratory diseases with molecular hydrogen.

CHAPTER 5

MASTERING MITOCHONDRIAL HEALTH

Mitochondria are organelles found in the cells of most eukaryotic organisms. They are often referred to as the "powerhouses of the cell" because they generate most of the cell's supply of adenosine triphosphate (ATP), which is used as a source of chemical energy.

5.1. Mitochondria by Numbers

A Deeper Dive

37 trillion cells: The human body is composed of approximately 37 trillion cells, each functioning as a unique unit with specific roles. Whether it's a neuron in your brain, a muscle fiber in your biceps, or a red blood cell delivering oxygen, every cell relies on mitochondria to meet its energy demands.

100's to 1000's of mitochondria per cell: While some cells, like skin cells, may contain only a few hundred mitochondria, energy-intensive cells such as muscle, brain, and liver cells can house thousands—up to 10,000 per cell. Heart cells, the powerhouses behind every beat, can host up to 100,000 mitochondria, given their massive energy requirements.

90% of cellular energy: Mitochondria are responsible for generating about 90% of the energy required by your cells through a process called oxidative phosphorylation. This energy is stored in the form of ATP (adenosine triphosphate), which cells use to perform vital functions like muscle contraction, neurotransmission, and detoxification.

100,000 heartbeats daily: Your heart doesn't take breaks, and its continuous pumping action requires a staggering amount of energy—about 100,000 beats every day! Mitochondria keep this essential muscle functioning, supplying energy for every contraction and relaxation.

2 billion ATP molecules per minute per mitochondrion: Mitochondria are ATP factories, and each one churns out an astonishing 2 billion molecules of ATP every minute. This energy currency fuels everything in your body—from blinking your eyes to running marathons.

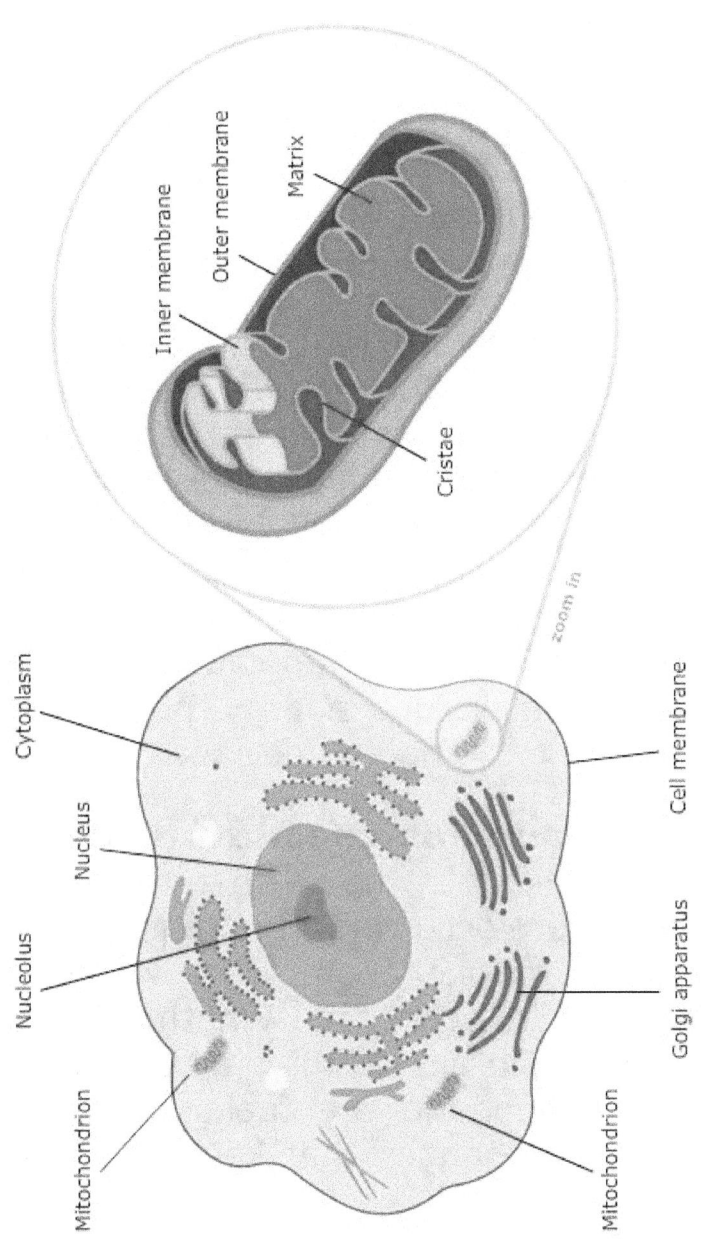

ATP production on a massive scale: The human body uses and recycles approximately 300–400 pounds of ATP every day, but it can only store a minuscule amount at any given time. Your mitochondria work overtime to ensure a constant supply, producing hundreds of quadrillions of ATP molecules daily to keep your cells functioning optimally.

Mitochondrial DNA: Unlike other cellular components, mitochondria have their own DNA, separate from the nuclear DNA. This double-stranded, circular mitochondrial DNA (mtDNA) encodes 13 essential proteins needed for energy production, making mitochondria semi-autonomous power plants. Damage to mtDNA, often caused by oxidative stress, can disrupt energy production and contribute to aging and disease.

1.8 quadrillion chemical reactions per second: That's how many biochemical reactions are occurring simultaneously in your cells, and most of them are powered by ATP from your mitochondria. Whether it's muscle contraction, brain activity, or cellular repair, your mitochondria are fueling the constant chemical exchanges that keep you alive and functioning.

Lifetime energy supply: In a single day, mitochondria produce an amount of ATP roughly equivalent to your body weight in energy molecules. Over a lifetime, that's enough energy to fuel thousands of miles of physical activity and countless hours of brain power.

Mitochondrial Networks: mitochondria aren't static; they form dynamic networks, constantly fusing and splitting in response to energy needs. This adaptability allows cells to respond to fluctuations in energy demand, repair damaged mitochondria, and optimize energy production based on metabolic activity.

The numbers tell an incredible story: mitochondria are central to not just life, but optimal health and performance. By maintaining mitochondrial health, you can fuel your body more efficiently, stave off disease, and slow down the aging process.

5.2. The Powerhouse Breakdown

5.2.1. What Makes Up the Mitochondria?

<u>Outer Membrane:</u> Think of this as a security gate. It's smooth and allows ions and small molecules to pass through using special proteins called porins.

Inner Membrane: This is the high-tech factory inside, full of folds called cristae where energy magic happens. It houses the electron transport chain and the engine for energy production—ATP synthase.

Matrix: This is the gel-like space inside the inner membrane, packed with the good stuff: mitochondrial DNA (mtDNA), ribosomes, and the key players in energy production, like the citric acid cycle (also known as the Krebs cycle).

Intermembrane Space: This gap between the inner and outer membranes is like the mitochondria's action-packed hallway, playing a crucial role in energy generation through the electron transport chain.

5.2.2. Mitochondria's Superpowers

ATP Production: This is mitochondria's main gig. Using a process called oxidative phosphorylation, they convert nutrients into ATP—the ultimate fuel your cells use to do, well, *everything*.

Metabolic Mastermind: Mitochondria regulate major pathways like the citric acid cycle, fatty acid breakdown, and amino acid metabolism.

<u>Cellular Suicide Squad:</u> Mitochondria control apoptosis, the process of programmed cell death, to get rid of cells that are damaged or no longer needed.

<u>Calcium Storage:</u> They help manage calcium levels, which is essential for cell signaling, muscle contractions, and more.

<u>Reactive Oxygen Species (ROS) Factory:</u> While making energy, mitochondria also produce ROS (byproduct molecules that can damage cells), which are important for signaling but can cause trouble if left unchecked.

5.2.3. Mitochondrial DNA

A Genetic Powerhouse

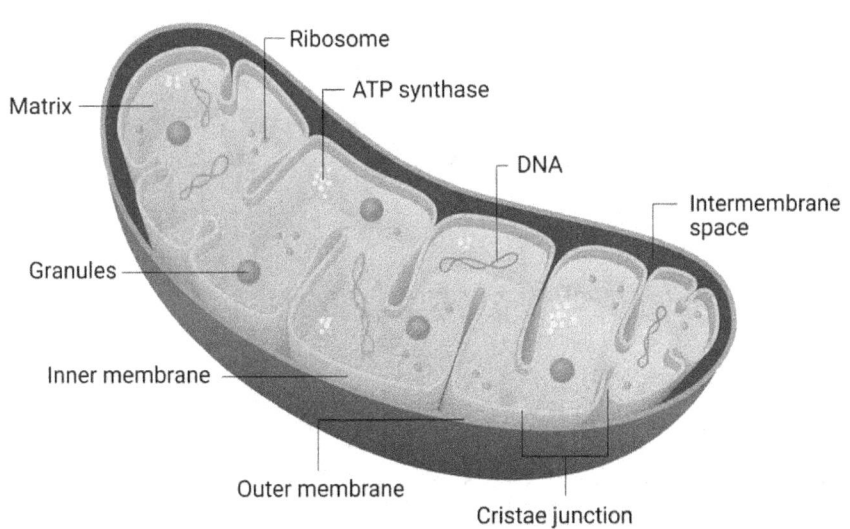

Unlike most organelles, mitochondria have their own DNA, called mitochondrial DNA (mtDNA). It's inherited from your mother and encodes key proteins for mitochondrial function. This mini genome is circular and much smaller than regular DNA.

5.2.4. Mitochondrial Dynamics

Always on the Move

Mitochondria are in a constant state of change, going through fusion (joining together) and fission (splitting apart). Fusion allows them to pool resources and share the wealth. Fission helps with cell division and discarding damaged parts. This constant remodeling keeps them working efficiently to meet your energy needs.

5.2.5. Energy Production - The Real MVP

Mitochondria produce energy via oxidative phosphorylation, a fancy term for a process that converts nutrients into ATP. Here's how:

Citric Acid Cycle (Krebs Cycle):

Takes place in the matrix, and breaks down fats, proteins, and carbs into high-energy molecules like NADH and $FADH_2$.

Electron Transport Chain (ETC):

Happens along the inner membrane. NADH and FADH$_2$ donate electrons, releasing energy that pumps protons (H$^+$) across the membrane, creating a proton gradient.

Chemiosmosis & ATP Synthesis:

Protons flow back through ATP synthase, turning the proton gradient into ATP. It's like a tiny generator inside your cells!

ATP Use:

ATP powers everything from muscle movement to protein creation and even cell division.

Efficiency & Heat Production:

Not all energy turns into ATP—some is released as heat, helping maintain your body temperature.

5.3. Mitochondrial Dysfunction

When Things Go Wrong

Mitochondrial dysfunction is like when your body's power plants start to break down.

Mitochondria, the tiny engines in your cells, are responsible for producing energy in the form of ATP. But when they malfunction, it's like a brownout in your cells, leading to fatigue, weakness, and even serious health problems.

From aging to cancer and chronic diseases, mitochondrial dysfunction plays a major role. It can happen because of genetic mutations, environmental toxins, poor diet, or even just stress. When these little powerhouses can't produce energy efficiently, you might feel it in your muscles, brain, and overall vitality.

Think of it this way: if your car's engine started sputtering, you'd lose speed and efficiency—well, that's what happens to your body when your mitochondria don't function properly. Luckily, lifestyle changes like better nutrition, exercise, and biohacking strategies can help get your cellular engines revving again.

5.3.1. Genetic Factors

Mitochondrial dysfunction and genetics are closely linked because your mitochondria have their own DNA! This tiny set of genetic instructions, passed down directly from your mother, controls much of how these cellular powerhouse's function. When there's a genetic mutation in this mitochondrial DNA (mtDNA), it can throw a wrench into the energy production process.

But that's not the only genetic factor at play. Most proteins your mitochondria need to work properly are coded by your nuclear DNA (the DNA you inherit from both parents). Mutations in these nuclear genes can also lead to mitochondrial dysfunction, disrupting energy production, and triggering various health issues.

This dysfunction can lead to a range of mitochondrial diseases, like Leigh syndrome or MELAS, which can cause symptoms such as muscle weakness, neurological problems, or even organ failure, especially in energy-hungry tissues like the brain and heart.

In short, when genetics go awry, your mitochondria can struggle to produce the energy your cells need, leading to serious health challenges.

_ However, the field of epigenetics has clearly established that we have the power to manipulate and alter our inherited genetics by up-regulating and down-regulating gene expression. Our genes do not define our fate. We do!

5.3.2. Toxemia Explained

So, what's toxemia? It literally means toxins in the blood, but let's break it down:

Our bodies are like non-stop factories, constantly building (anabolism) and breaking down cells (catabolism). The broken-down tissue is toxic, but in a healthy body, these toxins are flushed out. No harm, no foul!

But here's the catch: when we take in more toxins than our body can handle, they start to pile up in our blood and body. That's what we call toxemia, the accumulation of toxins in our body. These extra toxins are basically disease fuel.

Where do all these toxins come from? Check out these culprits:

Man-made food and drinks are loaded with artificial everything—sweeteners, colors, flavors, preservatives, gluten, high fructose corn syrup, GMOs, GMO rennet or FPC in cheeses, herbicides like glyphosate, pesticides, microplastics...you name it.

Seed oils, particularly those high in linoleic acid, have become a staple in modern diets, but they're hiding a dark side. Oils like soybean, corn, and sunflower are loaded with linoleic acid, an omega-6 fatty acid that, in excess, can lead to inflammation. While our bodies need a balance of omega-6 and omega-3 fatty acids, the modern diet is drowning in omega-6s, tipping the scales toward chronic inflammation. Over time, this inflammation can contribute to conditions like heart disease, obesity, and even cancer.

The real trouble with linoleic acid is how it behaves when heated. Seed oils break down easily under high temperatures, producing harmful compounds like aldehydes and oxidized fats, which are toxic to cells and can lead to oxidative stress. This kind of damage impacts everything from your gut health to the condition of your skin. So, while seed oils may seem harmless, their high linoleic acid content and instability under heat make them a toxic ingredient in many processed foods and fried dishes.

Medications— Medications, while designed to treat and manage health conditions, often come with a hidden cost—toxicity. Many pharmaceutical drugs are synthetic versions of natural compounds, but the chemical additives and artificial ingredients used to make them can introduce harmful toxins into the body. Over time, these toxins can accumulate, leading to unwanted side effects, liver strain, and even long-term health issues. Additionally, some medications can disrupt the body's natural processes, creating oxidative stress, damaging cells, and contributing to chronic inflammation. While they may offer short-term relief, their toxic load can have lasting consequences if not carefully managed.

Environmental exposure— In today's world, we're constantly surrounded by environmental toxins, from the air we breathe to the water we drink. Industrial pollution, car exhaust, and chemicals in cleaning products expose us to harmful substances like heavy metals, pesticides, and volatile organic compounds (VOCs).

Even our homes aren't safe havens, as common items like plastics, paints, and personal care products can release toxins that we inhale or absorb through the skin. These toxins accumulate in our bodies, disrupting cellular function and contributing to oxidative stress and systemic inflammation, which are known triggers for various health issues.

Xenoestrogens are synthetic compounds that mimic estrogen in the body, and they're sneaking into our lives through everyday products like plastics, pesticides, and personal care items. These hormone disruptors can wreak havoc on our endocrine system, leading to issues like hormonal imbalances, infertility, and even certain cancers. The problem with xenoestrogens is that they bind to estrogen receptors in our cells, overstimulating them and throwing off the body's natural hormone regulation. Over time, this can contribute to everything from weight gain and mood swings to more serious health concerns like breast and prostate cancer.

Additionally, modern life brings a new, invisible threat—electromagnetic radiation (EMR) from devices like smartphones, Wi-Fi routers, and microwaves. While often overlooked, EMR can affect our cells at a deep level, further compounding the impact of environmental toxins. As these toxins build up, they can impair organ function, disrupt hormones, and weaken the immune system, making it harder for our bodies to detoxify naturally.

EMR – The Invisible Threat

As we embrace smart tech and its endless conveniences, we often overlook the hidden health risks that come with it. A huge body of research shows that exposure to electromagnetic radiation (EMR) contributes to toxemia and even causes DNA damage. Want more details and hundreds of tips to protect yourself? Check out my bestseller, *EMR: The Invisible Threat – Strategies to Shield Yourself and Repair Your DNA.*

We've all heard of electromagnetic frequencies (EMFs), which are divided into ionizing (like X-rays) and non-ionizing (like your phone). While non-ionizing radiation was long considered safe, new research reveals that it can still cause cellular chaos.

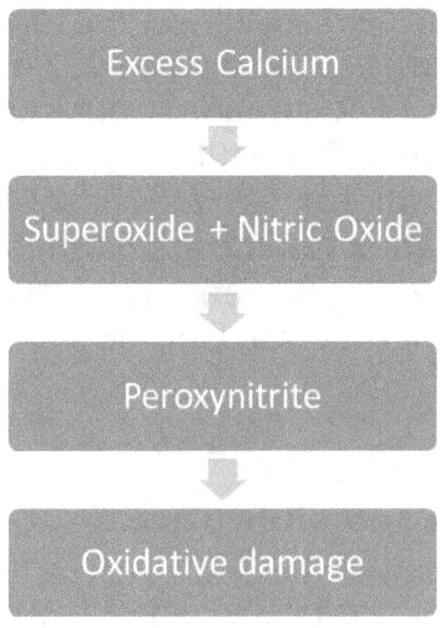

Here's how it works: EMR messes with tiny ion channels in our cells, flooding them with calcium. This overload leads to the creation of harmful compounds, like peroxynitrite, a nasty oxidant that sticks around longer than most free radicals, wreaking havoc on our DNA.

But don't panic—we've got a plan! Here's how to protect yourself from EMR's harmful effects:

- Minimize in-house exposure: Use filters, avoid wireless connections, and turn off Bluetooth when not needed.
- Shield your home: Protect yourself from EMR coming from neighbors, power lines, and smart meters.
- Shield yourself: Reduce exposure from your devices, use EMF-blocking products, and even try EMF protective clothing.
- Repair DNA damage: Since avoiding EMR completely isn't realistic, make sure to focus on repairing any DNA damage already done.

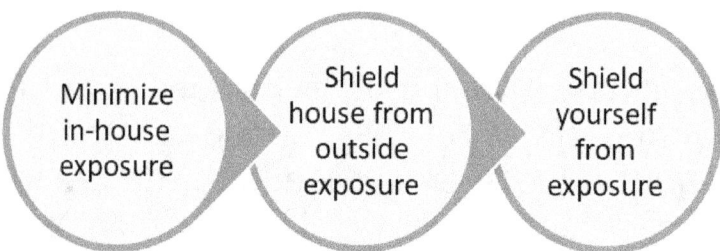

Take charge of your tech and your health with these simple steps! Check out the Resources page on my website for helpful information.

Stress and negative emotions— Stress and negative emotions don't just weigh on your mind; they take a serious toll on your body too. When we're stressed, the body goes into "fight or flight" mode, flooding the system with stress hormones like cortisol and adrenaline. While these hormones are great for helping us outrun a tiger, they're less helpful when triggered by daily annoyances. Chronic stress keeps these hormones elevated, which over time can lead to systemic inflammation, a key contributor to many chronic diseases. This constant state of high alert also impairs digestion, weakens the immune system, and slows down the body's detox processes, allowing harmful toxins to build up.

Negative emotions like anger, fear, and anxiety produce similar effects, adding a toxic load to the body. When we experience these emotions regularly, they create oxidative stress, leading to an overproduction of free radicals that damage cells and tissues. This toxic emotional state can contribute to everything from high blood pressure and heart disease to weakened immunity and poor mental health. The body and mind are deeply interconnected, so managing stress and fostering positive emotions can be as crucial to detoxification and health as diet and exercise!

What do these excess toxins do to our body?

These excess toxins are troublemakers. They steal electrons from healthy atoms, turning them into unstable, damaging free radicals. Your body's only defense? Antioxidants, which swoop in and donate electrons to calm the chaos.

With all those toxins running wild, your body goes into emergency mode, creating systemic inflammation. Even conventional medicine says 90% of diseases are caused by this chronic inflammation—think heart disease, arthritis, and more.

Bottom line: toxemia causes free radical damage and chronic inflammation, leading to disease. The solution? Reduce toxin intake, fight free radicals, and cut inflammation. Simple, right? You got this!

In Short, your mitochondria are your cells' energy factories, metabolic regulators, and even play a role in cell death and calcium storage. They are essential for life and health, but they need care and protection—whether it's from genetic mutations, environmental toxins, or oxidative stress. Keep them happy, and they'll keep you powered up!

5.3.3. Lifestyle Modifications

Let's dial it back to basics and refresh our approach to health with some simple yet powerful lifestyle tweaks. These tips are pulled straight from my book "The IZOD Method – Unleash Your Superpower," where I reveal the 7 foundations of optimal health in much more detail. Ready to get started? Let's dive in!

WATER: Imagine your body as a sophisticated plumbing system, with a circulatory system and lymphatic system working as your internal pipes. To keep these pipes clean and functioning smoothly, you need to drink plenty of pure, clean water.

Stagnation in your system can lead to problems, so make sure you're flushing out toxins regularly. For an extra boost, consider hydrogen-rich water, of course

AIR: Breathing isn't just about getting oxygen into your lungs; it's about doing it effectively. Most of us breathe too quickly and shallowly, which can make us less efficient. Instead, aim for slow, deep breaths: in through your nose for a count of 5, and out through your nose for a count of 6. And don't forget to go outside and enjoy the fresh, clean air. Indoor air can be stale and recycled, so soak up the benefits of nature whenever you can. To learn how to breathe properly, I suggest downloading the best APP, named The Source, a platform with the best breath masters in the world.

LIGHT: Sunlight is more than just a pleasant feeling; it's essential for vibrant health. Just as plants need sunlight to thrive, so do we. Exposure to natural light helps regulate your body's internal clock, stimulates all biological and physiological processes, and boosts your mood. So, get outside and enjoy the sunshine! Picture it as your daily energy recharges, giving you that extra pep in your step.

MOVEMENT: Think of your body as a dynamic, moving machine. Regular movement is key to avoiding stagnation and keeping your systems running smoothly. Instead of just hitting the gym for an hour, aim to stay active throughout the day. Take the stairs, go for walks, stretch regularly—basically, keep moving and grooving!

REST: Quality sleep is like your body's nightly maintenance session. To ensure you're getting restorative rest, avoid eating close to bedtime and incorporate a relaxation technique like visualization. Imagine walking through your next day and making positive choices—this can help calm your mind and prepare you for deep, refreshing sleep.

NUTRITION: Your diet is your body's fuel, so choose wisely. Aim to minimize the intake of processed foods and focus on nutrient-rich options. This means eating a variety of fruits, vegetables, carbs, lean proteins, and healthy fats. These foods not only keep your energy up but also help your body detoxify, fight inflammation, and support your immune system.

MINDSET: Your mind is like the superhero of your life, wielding immense power to shape your reality. The way you think, and feel can seriously impact your overall health and happiness. Cultivating a positive mindset is like giving yourself a turbo boost toward achieving your goals and dreams. When you believe in your potential and success, you're more likely to make those dreams come true.

I believe that your spirit picks your body with a special purpose in mind, and your mind is there to figure out how to live that purpose. But with around 14,000 messages bombarding us daily, it's no wonder things can get overwhelming! Your conscious mind takes in all this info through focused attention, like when you're reading or watching something. But most of the real magic happens in your subconscious mind—this is where your habits, emotions, and deep-seated beliefs hang out. This part of your mind connects you to the universe and its resources, and it's where your true potential resides.

Your ego, on the other hand, is a bit of a drama queen. It tries to protect you from distress based on what it knows, but it often gets in the way. To truly upgrade your mindset, you need to tap into the power of your subconscious mind and set your ego aside. Learn how to manage your feelings and emotions with strategies from "The IZOD Method – Unleash Your Superpower."

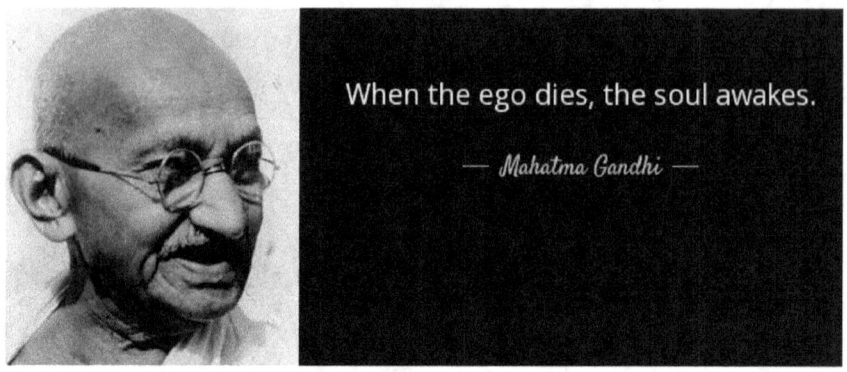

This seems like a lot of work, right? Not really, because you can stack these activities. For example, when you spend more time outdoors, you can get exposure to sunlight, breathe in fresh air and practice proper breathing or some mindfulness while walking (movement). In addition, you could take off your shoes and socks, and walk barefoot on grass or sand (beach) and get the benefits of grounding.

Grounding: Your Earthly Recharge

Grounding, or earthing if you're feeling fancy, is like plugging yourself into the planet's supercharger. Imagine it as your VIP pass to reconnect with Mother Nature's energy. Here's the lowdown on why kicking it with the Earth is a total game-changer:

What Is Grounding?

Think of grounding as your personal electric reset. By making skin-to-Earth contact—yes, that means ditching the shoes and feeling the grass or sand beneath your feet—you're tapping into the planet's natural electrons. These little guys are like the Earth's antioxidants, swooping in to zap away those pesky free radicals and bring your body's energy system back to Zen.

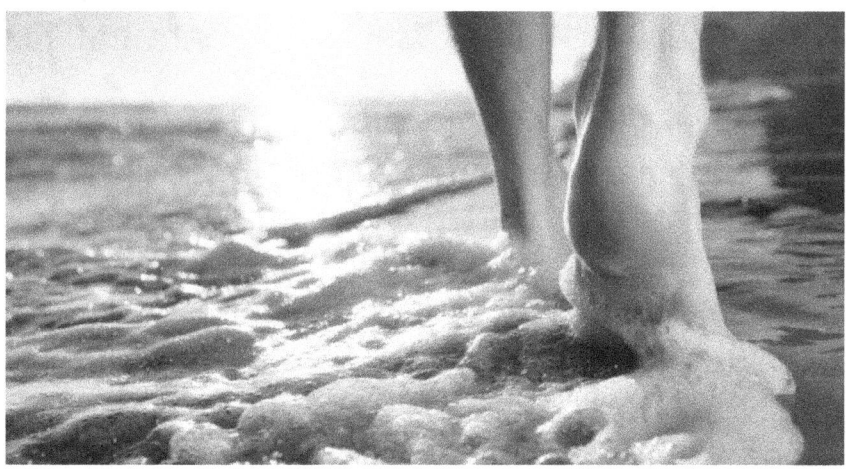

Why Bother?

In our tech-saturated world, we're like walking human antennas, picking up all sorts of electronic clutter. Grounding helps hit the reset button by reestablishing your connection to the Earth's natural vibe. The result? Reduced inflammation, better sleep, lower stress, and overall feel-good vibes. It's basically nature's way of giving you a high-five!

How to Get Grounded:

Grounding is as easy as pie—or should we say, as easy as taking off your shoes! Here's how to get started:

- <u>Barefoot Boogie:</u> Take a walk outside with your feet in direct contact with the Earth. It's like a free spa treatment for your soles!
- <u>Ground-Lounging:</u> Plop yourself down on the grass or sand, and just chill. Feel those good Earthy vibes soaking in.
- <u>Gardening:</u> Digging in the dirt not only connects you with the Earth but also makes you the coolest gardener in town.
- <u>Beach Bliss:</u> If you're near the coast, stroll along the shore or plant your butt in the sand for a double whammy of Earth and sea therapy.
- <u>Get Wet:</u> Swimming or playing around in open water such as lakes or the ocean also puts you in direct contact with Earth.

You will be moving, grounding and getting fresh air!

Health Perks:

Studies show that grounding can help dial down inflammation, boost your snooze game, and generally make you feel like a million bucks. It's like giving your body a natural tune-up without any weird gizmos or gadgets.

Daily Dose:

Just as the other 7 foundations, work grounding into your daily routine. Whether it's a barefoot morning jaunt or an evening grass session, these little Earth hugs can work wonders. So, ditch the shoes and give the Earth a high-five. Grounding is your shortcut to feeling fabulous, thanks to our planet's natural, no-fuss recharge. Let's get grounded and get glowing!

5.4. Boost Your Cells' Powerhouse with Molecular Hydrogen

Imagine if you could supercharge the tiny power plants inside your cells—the mitochondria—that keep your body running at full energy. Well, molecular hydrogen (H_2) is the new kid on the block when it comes to helping your mitochondria work better, faster, and longer. Ready to unlock the secret to better health? Let's break it down!

5.4.1. Fighting Oxidative Stress

Mitochondria work hard to produce energy, but they also create reactive oxygen species (ROS)—those nasty free radicals that can damage cells. Too many of them, and things start to go downhill.

- ✓ H_2 swoops in like a superhero, neutralizing only the worst of the ROS (like the destructive hydroxyl radicals) while leaving the good guys alone. It's like cleaning up a party without throwing out the pizza!
- ✓ Less ROS means your mitochondria stay safe and sound, pumping out energy without breaking down.

5.4.2. Boosting Energy Like a Power-Up

Your mitochondria are responsible for creating ATP, the energy currency your body runs on. But when they're tired or damaged, they can't produce as much, and you feel sluggish.

H_2 is the ultimate energy booster. It helps mitochondria work more efficiently, so you're producing top-quality ATP without all the waste. It's like giving your mitochondria a shot of espresso—more power, less crash!

5.4.3. Protecting the DNA That Runs the Show

Mitochondria have their own special DNA (mtDNA) that controls energy production. But this DNA is fragile and can easily be damaged by oxidative stress.

- ✓ H_2 acts like a shield, protecting mtDNA from free radicals and keeping your cellular engines running smoothly.
- ✓ With healthier mtDNA, your cells can keep firing on all cylinders, with fewer breakdowns along the way.

5.4.4. Building New Mitochondria (and Getting Rid of the Old Junk)

Sometimes, your cells need new mitochondria, or they need to take out the trash and get rid of the old, dysfunctional ones. H_2 can help with both.

- ✓ It promotes mitochondrial biogenesis, which is a fancy way of saying it helps

your cells make new, healthy mitochondria.
- ✓ It also encourages mitophagy—a process where damaged mitochondria get recycled. Out with the old, in with the new!

5.4.5. Cooling Inflammation to Keep Things Running Smoothly

When your mitochondria get stressed, they can trigger inflammation, which causes even more damage. It's like a vicious cycle of cellular chaos.

- ✓ H_2 steps in to calm the storm, reducing inflammatory signals and helping your mitochondria relax. It's like giving your cells a mini spa day!
- ✓ Less inflammation means happier mitochondria, and happier mitochondria means more energy for you.

5.4.6. Keeping the Mito Membrane Strong

The outer membrane of your mitochondria is like the border control of a country—it keeps things running smoothly. Damage this membrane, and it is game over for energy production.

- ✓ H_2 strengthens the mitochondrial membrane, making sure your cells can keep producing energy without any leaks or breakdowns.
- ✓ It's like upgrading the walls of your energy factory to titanium—sturdy, reliable, and tough to crack.

5.4.7. Brain Power - Protecting Neurons

Mitochondria don't just power your muscles—they're essential for brain health too. Mitochondrial dysfunction is a major player in neurodegenerative diseases like Alzheimer's and Parkinson's.

- ✓ H_2 helps neurons thrive by reducing oxidative stress and boosting mitochondrial function in brain cells. Think of it as a brain boost with long-term benefits.

The Bottom Line: Molecular hydrogen isn't just another health trend—it's like a personal trainer for your mitochondria. From boosting energy to keeping your cells younger for longer, H_2 is the secret weapon for unlocking the full potential of your cellular powerhouses. Want to feel more energized, think more clearly, and age more gracefully? H_2 might just be the answer.

CHAPTER 6

THE ART OF LONGEVITY & RADIANT BEAUTY

Who doesn't want to live longer, feel younger, and look better? We're all chasing that elusive fountain of youth—whether it's glowing skin, boundless energy, or simply staying sharp as we age. The good news? It's not just a dream anymore. With the right strategies, we can hack our health, slow down the aging clock, and look and feel our best for years to come. Let's dive into the secrets of living longer and thriving while looking fantastic!

6.1. H_2 Impact on Aging and Longevity

The impact of molecular hydrogen on the aging process is vast and biohackers benefit from the various positive effects hydrogen has within our cells and mitochondria. Molecular hydrogen has been studied for its potential effects on longevity and lifespan, largely due to its antioxidant, anti-inflammatory, and cellular protective properties.

Molecular hydrogen influences telomere attrition. Telomeres, the protective endcaps of our chromosomes in each cell, are susceptible to age-related deterioration. They play a critical role in cellular aging and longevity. Telomeres progressively shorten because of normal replication. When telomeres become too short, cells can no longer divide and enter a state known as senescence, which is linked to DNA damage, aging and various age-related diseases. Research indicates that H_2 has a universal anti-senescence impact, allowing cells and tissues continue to replicate and grow.

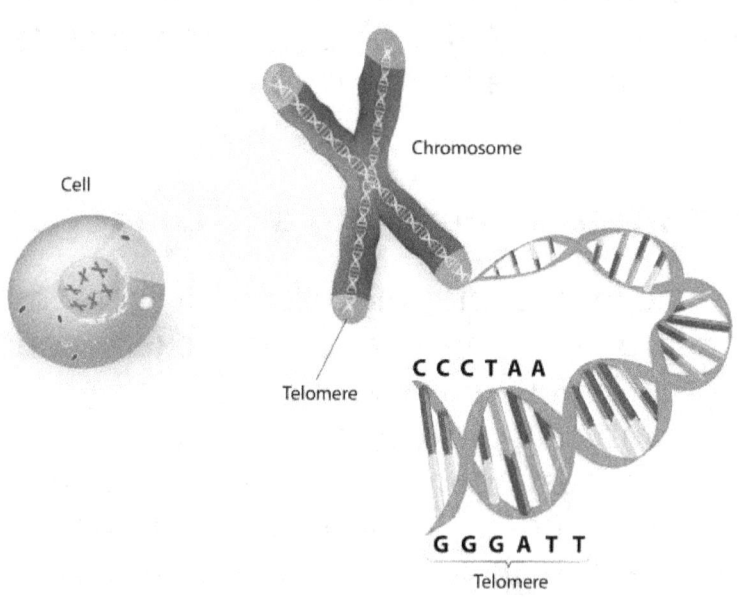

Furthermore, research indicates that the rate of telomere shortening may be accelerated by oxidative stress. Hence, we can infer that molecular hydrogen can also inhibit telomere shortening via its known action on inflammation and oxidative stress.

H_2 modulates mTOR, a multifunctional protein that regulates key cellular processes, including mRNA translation, protein synthesis, autophagy, transcription, and mitochondrial function. All these functions are involved in maintaining cellular homeostasis and modulating extended lifespan.

Our mitochondria, powerhouses for producing ATP required by every cell, have been shown to be promising therapeutic targets for influencing age-related disorders and longevity.

Molecular hydrogen prevents mitochondrial oxidative stress by directly neutralizing ROS and suppressing electron leakage. Molecular hydrogen regulates mitochondrial dynamics, modulates mitophagy, improves energy metabolism, and increases levels of ATP production. In addition, molecular hydrogen regulates apoptosis.

Molecular hydrogen is also known to affect our gut biome, a community of 100 trillion microbial cells that can enhance human metabolism, immune function, nutrition, and other physiological functions.

It restores the electrical potential of the gut when indicated, allowing the anaerobic bacteria to colonize.

In addition, molecular hydrogen improves DNA methylation, sleep quality, strength (lower body), general pain, brain metabolism indices, and antioxidant status.

6.1.1. Reduction of Oxidative Stress

Oxidative stress, caused by an imbalance between ROS and the body's antioxidant defenses, is a key factor in aging and age-related diseases. H_2 selectively neutralizes harmful ROS, particularly hydroxyl radicals (•OH), without disrupting the beneficial ROS involved in normal cellular functions.

By reducing oxidative stress, H_2 can help protect cells from damage, which may contribute to improved health and potentially increased lifespan.

6.1.2. Anti-inflammatory Properties

Chronic or systemic inflammation, or "inflammaging," is associated with many age-related diseases, including cardiovascular disease, neurodegenerative conditions, and metabolic disorders. H_2 has been shown to reduce the levels of pro-inflammatory cytokines (e.g., TNF-α, IL-6, IL-1β) and promote anti-inflammatory cytokines (e.g., IL-10).

By reducing systemic inflammation, H_2 can help prevent or delay the onset of age-related diseases, potentially contributing to a longer, healthier life.

6.1.3. Protection Against Age-Related Diseases

Support of Cellular Health:

H_2's antioxidant and anti-inflammatory effects can help protect against various age-related diseases, such as cardiovascular disease, neurodegenerative disorders, and metabolic conditions. By mitigating the damage and dysfunction associated with these diseases, H_2 may improve overall health and longevity.

Prevention of Cellular Damage:

H_2 helps protect cells from oxidative damage and supports cellular repair mechanisms, which can be crucial in preventing diseases that commonly affect older individuals.

6.1.4. Support of Mitochondrial Function

Mitochondrial dysfunction is a hallmark of aging and is associated with reduced energy production and increased oxidative stress. H_2 supports mitochondrial function by reducing oxidative damage and promoting mitochondrial biogenesis (the creation of new mitochondria).

Improved mitochondrial health can enhance cellular energy production, reduce fatigue, and support overall cellular function, which can contribute to longevity.

6.1.5. Enhancement of Cellular Repair Mechanisms

Autophagy and DNA Repair:

H_2 may influence cellular repair processes, such as autophagy (the removal of damaged proteins and organelles) and DNA repair mechanisms. These processes are crucial for maintaining cellular health and function, particularly in the context of aging.

By enhancing these repair mechanisms, H_2 can help maintain cellular integrity and function, potentially contributing to a longer lifespan.

6.1.6. Improvement of Cognitive Function

Neuroprotection:

Cognitive decline is a significant aspect of aging, with conditions such as Alzheimer's disease and other forms of dementia becoming more common. H_2's neuroprotective effects, including its ability to reduce oxidative stress and inflammation in the brain, may help maintain cognitive function and prevent neurodegenerative diseases.

By supporting brain health, H_2 may contribute to a higher quality of life in older age.

6.1.7. Telomere protection

Reduction of Oxidative Stress:

Oxidative stress accelerates telomere shortening by causing damage to the DNA and telomere regions. H_2's antioxidant properties help neutralize reactive oxygen species (ROS), particularly the hydroxyl radical (•OH), which can damage telomeric DNA.

By reducing oxidative stress, H_2 may help protect telomeres from damage and potentially slow the rate of telomere shortening.

Support of Cellular Health:

H_2's ability to reduce oxidative stress and inflammation can contribute to overall cellular health. Healthy cells are less likely to experience accelerated telomere shortening due to reduced cellular damage and stress.

By supporting cellular health, H_2 may indirectly help maintain telomere length and function.

Influence on Cellular Senescence:

Cellular senescence is associated with shortened telomeres and is a key feature of aging. H_2 may help reduce the factors that contribute to cellular senescence, such as oxidative stress and inflammation.

This reduction in senescence could help preserve telomere length and improve overall cellular function.

Potential Impact on Telomerase Activity:

Telomerase is an enzyme that can add DNA sequence repeats to telomeres, counteracting the effects of telomere shortening. Although H_2's direct impact on telomerase activity is not well-studied, its overall effects on cellular health and oxidative stress might influence telomerase activity indirectly.

If H_2 supports a healthier cellular environment, it may create conditions more favorable for telomerase activity and telomere maintenance.

In short, molecular hydrogen may have a beneficial impact on telomeres primarily through its antioxidant properties, which help reduce oxidative stress that accelerates telomere shortening. By protecting cells from oxidative damage and supporting overall cellular health, H_2 could indirectly contribute to the maintenance of telomere length and function.

While direct research on H_2 and telomeres is limited, the broader evidence supporting antioxidants in telomere maintenance suggests that H_2 might play a positive role in preserving telomere health and potentially influencing aging processes.

Further research is needed to establish a direct connection between H_2 and telomere dynamics and to understand its full potential in promoting longevity and health.

6.2. BIOHACKING OUR DNA

Relatively recent scientific research shows that we have an innate DNA repair mechanism. Understanding this repair mechanism and its essential components is the key to a better approach in reversing DNA damage from various environmental toxins, electromagnetic radiation (EMR) and other sources.

6.2.1. ARTD1 Repair System

ADP-ribosyltransferase diphtheria toxin-like 1 (ARTD1), formerly known as poly ADP-ribose polymerase (PARP) is a family of 17 enzymes that function as DNA damage sensors and signaling molecules. They bind to damaged DNA, create a matrix, and allow specific DNA repair enzymes to repair the damage.

This DNA repair process requires fuel. This fuel is nicotinamide adenine dinucleotide or NAD+. Our bodies can repair minimal to moderate DNA damage through this process but when moderate to severe DNA damage occurs (as with the exposure to EMR), cells become NAD+ depleted, which stops the repair system (no fuel), resulting in cell death.

In addition, NAD+ depletion affects our mitochondria and ATP (energy) production.

NAD+ depletion consequently depletes sirtuins in our body. Sirtuins are known as our longevity proteins. Sirtuins need NAD+ to function and without sirtuins, aging is significantly accelerated.

Another consequence of activating the repair system is the activation of pro-inflammatory pathways.

To successfully repair DNA damage, we then need to make sure we have an adequate supply of NAD+ so we don't run out of fuel, and that we use nutrients that fight oxidation and inflammation.

6.2.2. NAD+ and NADPH

NAD+, or nicotinamide adenine dinucleotide, is a critical coenzyme found in every cell in our body, and it is involved in hundreds of metabolic processes. NAD+ has two general sets of reactions in the human body: helping turn nutrients into energy as a key player in metabolism and working as a helper molecule for proteins that regulate other cellular functions. These processes are incredibly important and include:

- ✓ DNA repair
- ✓ Mitochondrial function
- ✓ Maintaining chromosomal integrity
- ✓ Gene expression
- ✓ Epigenetic modifications
- ✓ Posttranslational modifications
- ✓ Calcium signaling

Some of the proteins that regulate these processes are called sirtuins, which regulate cell health, including cellular resistance to stressful conditions and aging. Sirtuins require NAD+ to function. However, NAD+ is reduced and converted to NADH once it transports electrons. Thus, our bodies need to continually synthesize NAD+. Herein lies the dilemma. Our bodies produce less and less NAD+ as we age, and NAD+ is depleted with increased toxic exposure since our innate repair system for DNA damage uses high amounts of NAD+ as fuel.

Scientists suggest that declining levels of NAD+ are associated with signs of aging and age-related illnesses. Research shows that restoring NAD+ levels and keeping NADPH levels high are essential to maintain cellular health.

NAD+ levels currently cannot simply be measured in a laboratory. Normal levels for healthy people, age 30 or younger are 40ng/ml while these levels drop progressively as we age and reach 1 ng/ml at age 80. Keeping your NAD+ levels high can be done as follows:

- ✓ Low EMR-lifestyle. EMR depletes NAD+ by activating the repair process that uses NAD+ as fuel.

- ✓ Adequate rest and sleep allow the repair, regeneration, and renewal of damaged tissue. Eat dinner early in the evening and then refrain from foods and snacks so digestion can occur prior to sleeping. This practice also prevents energy from food being stored as fat, which requires NADPH (see below).

- ✓ Supplement with tryptophan, an amino acid that can produce NAD+ in small amounts. Tryptophan is also a precursor for serotonin and melatonin, which may therefore improve sleep and mood.

- ✓ A heathy diet that limits toxins and combats toxemia and inflammation.

- ✓ Niacin is a precursor for NAD+. Take 20-30mg daily.

- ✓ Supplement with NMN or even better niacinamide (250mg/day).

- ✓ NQO1 is the enzyme that converts NADH to NAD+ and can be increased by heat exposure such as with a near-infrared sauna or photodynamic therapy (PDT). These therapies therefore increase NAD+ but they also help eliminate toxins (perspiration) and energize our mitochondria. NQO1 also activates the Nrf2 pathway (see later).

- ✓ Implement high-intensity exercises or resistance training. Both forms of exercise indirectly increase NAD+ and slow down the age-dependent decline in NAD+.

- ✓ Another way to increase NAD+ according to Dr. Mercola is Blood Flow Restriction Training which uses low weights with high repetitions. For more information, visit BFR.mercola.com.

NADPH is another coenzyme, part of the NAD family. NADPH is the actual battery of our cells. NADPH provides a reservoir of electrons (from hydrogen) and therefore can donate a continuous supply of electrons to antioxidants. This way, antioxidants such as vitamin C, D and E can keep neutralizing free radicals and minimize damage from oxidative stress. Without NADPH, vitamin C and other antioxidants become oxidized and useless.

NADPH recharges the antioxidants inside the cell. Remember that many antioxidants, including vitamin C, are charged and cannot enter the cell.

As you can see, it's important to have antioxidants but it's even more important to sustain adequate levels of NADPH so we can recharge the antioxidants for more effective repair of DNA damage and oxidative stress.

This is how you can increase NADPH levels in your body:

- ✓ Low EMR-lifestyle. EMR depletes NAD+ by activating the repair process that uses NAD+ as fuel. NAD+ is required for NADPH synthesis. In addition, NADPH oxidase (NOX), an enzyme that breaks down NADPH, is activated by EMR via the calcium influx into the cell and increases superoxide production which combines with nitric oxide to form peroxynitrite, a highly reactive free radical.

- ✓ Molecular hydrogen (H_2) inhibits the activation of NOX.

- ✓ Pau D'arco tea contains beta-lapachone which acts as a catalyst for NAD. This nutty-tasting tea (or supplement) promotes NAD activity, mitochondrial health, and regulates genetic anti-aging processes. Drink as tea or use as a smoothie base or mix with coconut milk or oil.

- ✓ Refrain from eating 3-4 hours before going to sleep. The enzymes used to store energy from food as fat use large amounts of NADPH.

Impact of H_2

H_2 inhibits NOX but only when NOX is excessively activated, to preserve a necessary balance. NOX has several important functions, including assisting the white blood cells in destroying pathogens such as viruses and bacteria, cell signaling, and regulating gene expression.

Besides increasing NADPH levels, H_2 also

can protect our DNA, RNA, mitochondria, proteins, and cell membranes from oxidative damage.

H_2 is the smallest molecule and lightest element in the universe and is not charged which allows it to easily cross cell membranes and enter the cell. H_2 is highly bioavailable (easily absorbed). Therefore, H_2 is effective in mitigating damaging effects of oxidative stress inside the cell and subcellular structures.

H_2 also stimulates the NRF2 pathway.

The NAD Family

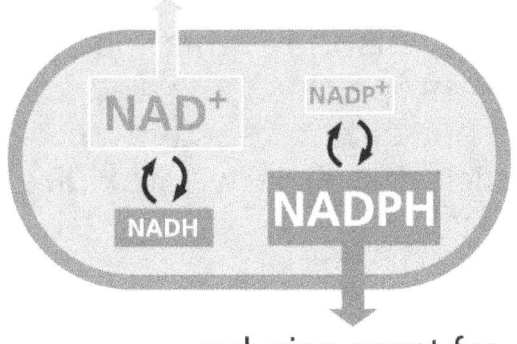

The NAD (nicotinamide adenine dinucleotide) family includes NAD^+ and its reduced form, NADH, as well as related molecules like $NADP^+$ and NADPH. These molecules play critical roles in cellular metabolism, energy production, and redox reactions.

Research into molecular hydrogen (H_2) and its effects on the NAD family is still in its early stages, but there are several ways H_2 might influence NAD metabolism and related processes:

Reduction of Oxidative Stress:

Impact on Redox Balance:

NAD^+ and NADH are central to redox reactions, where NAD^+ is reduced to NADH and NADH is oxidized back to NAD^+. Oxidative stress can disrupt this balance. H_2's antioxidant properties help reduce oxidative stress by neutralizing reactive oxygen species (ROS), which can otherwise oxidize NADH or reduce NAD^+.

By maintaining redox balance, H_2 can support the proper functioning of NAD-dependent enzymes and metabolic pathways.

Support of Cellular Energy Production:

Role in Metabolism:

NAD^+ is essential for glycolysis, the citric acid cycle, and oxidative phosphorylation, all of which are crucial for ATP production. H_2 may indirectly support these processes by reducing oxidative stress and inflammation, which can otherwise impair mitochondrial function and NAD^+ utilization.

Improved cellular health and reduced oxidative stress can enhance the efficiency of NAD^+-dependent energy production pathways.

Influence on NAD-Dependent Enzymes:

Sirtuins and PARPs:

NAD^+ is a cofactor for sirtuins and poly (ADP-ribose) polymerases (PARPs), both of which are involved in regulating cellular stress responses, DNA repair, and promoting longevity. H_2's antioxidant and anti-inflammatory effects can support the optimal functioning of these NAD-dependent enzymes.

By reducing oxidative damage and inflammation, H_2 may help maintain the activity of sirtuins and PARPs, which are important for cellular health and longevity.

Impact on Cellular Repair Mechanisms:

DNA Repair and Longevity:

PARPs, which use NAD^+, play a key role in DNA repair processes. H₂ may support DNA repair by reducing oxidative damage and enhancing the availability of NAD^+ for PARP activity.

By promoting effective DNA repair, H₂ can contribute to cellular longevity and resilience against stress.

Potential Influence on NAD+ Synthesis:

NAD+ Precursors:

NAD^+ can be synthesized from precursors like niacin (vitamin B3) and tryptophan. While direct evidence of H₂ influencing NAD^+ synthesis is limited, reducing oxidative stress and supporting overall cellular health could improve the efficiency of NAD^+ synthesis and utilization.

Experimental Evidence:

Animal and Cell Studies:

While specific studies on H₂ and NAD are limited, research on antioxidants and cellular redox balance provides indirect evidence that

H_2 might support NAD^+-dependent processes by mitigating oxidative stress.

Human Research:

Clinical studies exploring the effects of H_2 on metabolism and cellular health may offer insights into its impact on NAD metabolism and related pathways.

In short, molecular hydrogen may influence the NAD family through its antioxidant and anti-inflammatory effects, supporting redox balance, energy production, and the functioning of NAD-dependent enzymes like sirtuins and PARPs. While direct research on H_2 and NAD is limited, the broader evidence suggesting that antioxidants can benefit NAD metabolism indicates that H_2 might play a supportive role in maintaining cellular health and longevity. Further research is needed to clarify the specific interactions between H_2 and NAD metabolism and to understand its potential benefits fully.

6.2.3. Nrf2 Pathway

The Nrf2 pathway is the master regulator of responses to oxidative damage caused by free radicals, mitochondrial dysfunction, and systemic inflammation.

The body only calls this pathway into action when free radical damage needs to be reduced. Nrf2 stimulates our DNA to activate 100's of genes, including antioxidants and enzymes that respond to toxic chemicals, stress, and free radical damage.

Nrf2 also increases NADPH and is considered essential in living a longer and healthier life.

Nrf2 stimulates autophagy (self-eating) and is especially effective when fasting.

Antioxidants and polyphenols in fruits and vegetables stimulate the Nrf2 pathway. Remember that it's always better that we get our antioxidants from whole foods versus supplements. Too many antioxidants may deplete important free radicals that act as scavengers.

Research shows that the following list of foods and their active ingredient(s) activate the Nrf2 pathway:

- ✓ Turmeric (curcumin)
- ✓ Green tea (EGCG, Fisetin, Rutin)
- ✓ Black tea, Buckwheat (Rutin)
- ✓ Grapes, blueberries, dark chocolate, pistachios (Resveratrol)

- ✓ Strawberries, apple, chamomile tea (Fisetin)
- ✓ Apple peel (polyphenols)
- ✓ Pomegranate peel (polyphenols)
- ✓ Broccoli (sulforaphane, isothiocyanates, quercetin)
- ✓ Cabbage (isothiocyanates)
- ✓ Red onions, capers, berries (quercetin)
- ✓ Garlic, onion, chives, leeks (sulfur)
- ✓ Tomatoes, guava, and watermelon (lycopene)
- ✓ Beans, oregano, thyme, and peppermint (terpenes)
- ✓ Cannabis and CBD oils (terpenes)
- ✓ Krill, microalgae (astaxanthin)
- ✓ Fish oil (omega-3, DHA, EPA)
- ✓ Vitamin D
- ✓ H_2
- ✓ Melatonin

Moderate exercise also activates the Nrf2 pathway.

Constant stimulation of the Nrf2 pathway would be counterproductive as balance in the body is essential.

The Nrf2 pathway is essential is keeping toxemia in check as it removes toxic chemicals, neutralizes free radicals, and fights systemic inflammation while simultaneously assisting in the repair of DNA damage through NADPH stimulation and autophagy.

6.2.4. Magnesium Magic

Magnesium is an essential mineral in cell repair, cell function, RNA synthesis, and DNA synthesis.

Magnesium is also a calcium channel blocker. Therefore, magnesium can reduce the amount of superoxide and peroxynitrite produced in our body with EMR exposure.

Foods containing fair amounts of magnesium:

- ✓ Avocados
- ✓ Almonds
- ✓ Brazil nuts
- ✓ Cashews
- ✓ Peanuts
- ✓ Spinach
- ✓ Broccoli
- ✓ Squash seeds
- ✓ Pumpkin seeds
- ✓ Hemp seeds
- ✓ Chia seeds
- ✓ Edamame
- ✓ Quinoa
- ✓ Coconut milk

- ✓ Figs
- ✓ Lima beans
- ✓ Swiss chard
- ✓ Okra
- ✓ Beet greens
- ✓ Bananas
- ✓ Dark chocolate (85% cocoa)
- ✓ Brown rice
- ✓ Oatmeal
- ✓ Black beans
- ✓ Tuna
- ✓ Mackerel
- ✓ Salmon
- ✓ Yoghurt or Kefir

Be aware that nuts and seeds may contain linoleic acid.

I recommend 500-1000mg of elemental magnesium per day. Be aware that the elemental magnesium is the magnesium available to our body and usually is only 8-15% of the total amount of magnesium.

Supplements use various forms of magnesium, including citrate, malate, glycinate, threonate, and oxide. I don't recommend magnesium oxide because it's poorly absorbed by our body. I suggest you take a combination or one of the following:

- ✓ Citrate: high bioavailability and citrate helps bind oxalates (prevent or helps with oxalate crystals and kidney stones).

- ✓ Malate: high bioavailability and helps with muscle tightness / spasms.

- ✓ Glycinate: glycine helps increase NADPH and helps with connective tissue strength.

- ✓ Threonate: threonate has the highest bioavailability. Threonate also helps magnesium pass the blood-brain barrier which helps increase magnesium levels in the brain. It is said to help with depression and GI discomfort.

I personally opt for the Threonate form of magnesium, but you can also consider taking a magnesium supplement that contains a combination of these various forms of magnesium such as Magnesium Breakthrough by BioOptimizers.

My Fullscript page has a few great options for you. Check it out by clicking the link on the bottom of my homepage at MVTonline.com

6.2.5. Nitric Oxide

Nitric oxide production is essential for overall health because it allows blood, nutrients, and oxygen to travel to every part of our body effectively and efficiently.

In fact, a limited capacity to produce nitric oxide is associated with heart disease, diabetes, and erectile dysfunction.

Nitric oxide is synthesized by many cell types involved in immunity and inflammation. The principal enzyme involved is the inducible type-2 isoform of nitric oxide synthase (NOS-2), which produces high-level sustained nitric oxide.

Nitric Oxide is important as a toxic defense molecule against infectious organisms. It also regulates the functional activity, growth, and death of many immune and inflammatory cell types including macrophages, T lymphocytes, antigen-presenting cells, mast cells, neutrophils, and natural killer cells.

Fortunately, there are many ways to maintain optimal levels of nitric oxide in our body.

Vegetables are good sources of nitrates, which help form nitric oxide in our body. Consuming nitrate-rich vegetables improves heart health and exercise performance.

Vegetables with high in nitrates include:

- ✓ Red spinach
- ✓ Cress
- ✓ Celery
- ✓ Chervil
- ✓ Lettuce
- ✓ Beetroot
- ✓ Spinach
- ✓ Arugula
- ✓ Garlic
- ✓ Kale

Also, citrus fruits including oranges, lemon, limes, and pomegranate are loaded with potent antioxidants that can protect our cells against damage and preserve nitric oxide. Nuts and seeds are high in arginine, an amino acid needed to produce nitric oxide. But be aware of the linoleic acid levels in certain nuts and seeds.

Nitric oxide is an unstable molecule that degrades quickly in the bloodstream, so it must be constantly replenished. One way to increase its stability and limit its breakdown is by consuming antioxidants.

Several supplements are marketed as "nitric oxide boosters." These supplements do not contain nitric oxide itself, but they include ingredients that help form nitric oxide in our body. Two of the most used ingredients are L-arginine and L-citrulline.

Exercise and/or movement gets our blood pumping, largely because it improves endothelial function. Endothelium is the thin layer of cells that line the blood vessels. These cells naturally produce nitric oxide, which keeps blood vessels healthy.

Insufficient nitric oxide production results in endothelium dysfunction, which can contribute to atherosclerosis, high blood pressure, and other risk factors for heart disease.

Mouthwash destroys bacteria in our mouth that can contribute to the growth of cavities and other dental diseases. Unfortunately, mouthwash kills all types of bacteria, including the beneficial ones that help produce nitric oxide.

Special bacteria in the mouth convert nitrate to nitric oxide. In fact, humans cannot produce nitric oxide from nitrate without these bacteria. This leads to a decrease in nitric oxide production and, in some instances, an increase in blood pressure.

The detrimental effects of mouthwash on nitric oxide production may even contribute to the development of diabetes, which is characterized by malfunctions in insulin production or action. This is because nitric oxide also regulates insulin, which helps cells utilize the energy obtained from food after it's digested. Without nitric oxide, insulin cannot work properly.

Sun exposure does more than just light up your day—it also plays a key role in boosting your cellular health by releasing nitric oxide. When UV rays hit your skin, they prompt the production of nitric oxide, which helps improve blood flow and oxygen delivery to cells. This increased circulation supports cellular energy, efficiency, and overall function, making your cells more resilient and effective.

Nitric oxide also helps reduce oxidative stress, keeping your cells protected and promoting better overall health, so catching some rays can be a great way to boost your vitality!

<u>Breathwork</u>, especially through nasal breathing, is a natural way to boost nitric oxide (NO) levels in the body, which has a significant impact on cellular health. When you breathe through your nose, the nasal passages release nitric oxide, a powerful molecule that helps improve oxygen delivery and blood circulation. This enhanced oxygen flow supports better energy production at the cellular level, making your cells more efficient

Just as deficiency of nitric oxide can lead to disease, too much can also cause disease. Nitric oxide may damage brain cells leading to neurodegenerative diseases like Parkinson disease, Alzheimer disease, Huntington disease, and amyotrophic lateral sclerosis. Higher than normal levels of exhaled nitric oxide generally mean your airways are inflamed — a sign of asthma. An oral exhaled nitric oxide value of more than 40 parts per billion for adults and more than 25 parts per billion for children and adolescents is considered elevated.

We also know that nitric oxide combines with superoxide to form peroxynitrite, which produces harmful carbonate free radicals. We need to control the superoxide production in our body to prevent the formation of peroxynitrite.

6.2.6. Methylene Blue – The Blue Wonder

Methylene blue is not just your average dye. It's a synthetic marvel with the chemical formula $C_{16}H_{18}ClN_3S$, and it's been making waves since its creation in the late 19th century. Originally whipped up for textile dyeing, it soon found its way into the world of medicine and science. Picture it as a deep blue powder that turns water into a sapphire solution—it's a color statement and a scientific tool all in one.

Environmental and Educational Uses:

Eco-Friendly Investigator: Methylene blue is a hero in environmental science, used to trace pollutants and monitor water quality. It's like a detective for our planet's health.

Classroom Companion: In education, it's a favorite for staining slides in microscopy. It helps students see cell structures clearly, turning abstract concepts into tangible visuals.

Medical Marvel

Diagnostic Dynamo: In the medical realm, methylene blue shines as a diagnostic hero. It's used to stain tissue samples, helping pathologists see the finer details of cellular structures. Think of it as a highlighter for your cells.

Antiseptic Ace: It's also had a stint as an antiseptic and anti-parasitic agent. While it's not the go-to treatment these days, it's still employed in specific scenarios like treating methemoglobinemia—a condition where your blood isn't delivering oxygen properly.

Surgical Sidekick: Surgeons use it to track fluids and identify tissue damage during operations, making it a trusty tool in the OR.

Neuroprotective Potential: Methylene blue might have a few tricks up its sleeve for brain health too. Researchers are exploring its role in neuroprotection, particularly for conditions like Alzheimer's and Parkinson's disease. Its ability to support mitochondrial function and reduce oxidative damage could help keep those brain cells healthier for longer.

Recently, methylene blue had garnered attention for its fascinating interactions with mitochondria, the energy powerhouses of our cells.

Mitochondrial Marvel

Here's where things get exciting. Methylene blue is emerging as a potential game-changer for mitochondrial health. Mitochondria, often called the powerhouses of our cells, are crucial for generating energy. Methylene blue acts like a turbocharger for these little energy factories, boosting their efficiency and protecting them from oxidative stress. It enhances mitochondrial function, which can lead to better overall cellular health and energy production.

Here's a closer look at how it affects mitochondrial function:

Enhancing Mitochondrial Respiration

Methylene blue enhances mitochondrial respiration, the process by which cells produce energy. It helps facilitate electron transport within the mitochondria, boosting the efficiency of ATP (adenosine triphosphate) production, which is crucial for cellular energy.

Reducing Oxidative Stress

Mitochondria are susceptible to oxidative stress, which can damage cellular components and contribute to aging and disease. Methylene blue acts as an antioxidant, reducing oxidative damage by neutralizing free radicals. This helps maintain mitochondrial health and function.

Improving Mitochondrial Function

Research suggests that methylene blue can improve mitochondrial function by stabilizing the mitochondrial membrane and enhancing the efficiency of the electron transport chain. This means that mitochondria can generate energy more effectively and with less waste.

Supporting Mitochondrial Repair

Methylene blue may aid in mitochondrial repair by promoting the production of protective factors and reducing inflammation. This support helps maintain mitochondrial integrity and function over time.

Potential Benefits in Neurodegenerative Diseases

Given that many neurodegenerative diseases are linked to mitochondrial dysfunction, methylene blue's mitochondrial-enhancing properties have been explored for potential therapeutic benefits. It might help in conditions like Alzheimer's disease and Parkinson's disease by supporting mitochondrial health and reducing cellular damage.

Modulating Mitochondrial Dynamics

Methylene blue may influence mitochondrial dynamics, which involves the balance between mitochondrial fission (splitting) and fusion (joining). Proper regulation of these processes is vital for maintaining healthy mitochondrial function and overall cellular health.

Cellular Energy Boost

By improving mitochondrial efficiency, methylene blue may help boost overall cellular energy levels. This can enhance physical performance, reduce fatigue, and support overall vitality.

In short, methylene blue's impact on mitochondria makes it a compelling area of study for enhancing cellular energy and combating oxidative stress.

While the potential benefits are exciting, it's essential to use it with caution and under medical supervision, as high doses or improper use can lead to side effects. Always consult with a healthcare provider before starting any new treatments or supplements.

6.2.7. The Bucky Ball - Carbon Superstar

The Marvel of Molecular Geometry

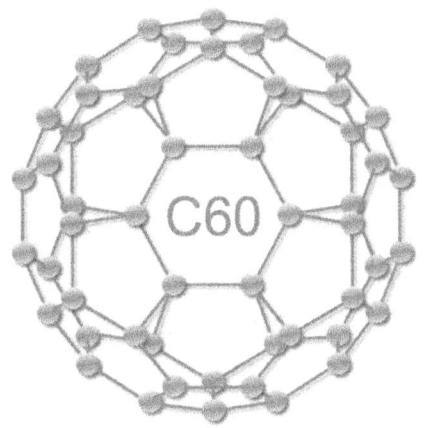

Meet C60, affectionately known as Buckminsterfullerene or the bucky ball—a molecule that looks like the fanciest soccer ball you've ever seen. Composed of 60 carbon atoms arranged in a geometric pattern, this molecular marvel is not just a sight to behold but a powerhouse of potential. Discovered in 1985, C60 resembles a truncated icosahedron, a shape with hexagons and pentagons reminiscent of a geodesic dome.

The Science of C60

Antioxidant Avenger: C60 is like a superhero for your cells. Its structure allows it to act as an incredibly powerful antioxidant, swooping in to neutralize harmful free radicals, particularly superoxide. Superoxide is a rogue free radical known for wreaking havoc in cells, and C60 is its nemesis. By mopping up these free radicals, C60 helps protect cells from oxidative stress and damage.

Mitochondrial Magic: Think of C60 as a VIP guest at the mitochondrial party. Due to its ability to absorb protons and its positive charge, C60 can slip through the mitochondrial membrane with ease. Once inside, it works diligently to decrease free radical production. This means your mitochondria—those tiny energy factories in your cells—are less burdened by oxidative stress and can function more efficiently, boosting your energy levels and overall cellular health.

Anti-Inflammation Dynamo: Beyond its antioxidant prowess, C60 is a systemic inflammation fighter. Chronic inflammation is a silent troublemaker behind many health issues, and C60 acts as a powerful ally in reducing inflammation throughout the body. By keeping inflammation in check, it helps combat various health conditions and supports overall well-being.

Aging and Longevity Legend

C60 isn't just about fighting off villains; it's also about making you feel and look young. In a groundbreaking 2012 study, French scientists fed rats C60 dissolved in olive oil, and the results were astonishing—these rats almost doubled their lifespan! While it's a stretch to say C60 is the fountain of youth, its potential to slow aging and enhance longevity is incredibly promising.

Health Heroics

Neuroprotective Ninja: C60 may also play a role in brain health. It's being researched for its potential to prevent neurodegenerative diseases like Alzheimer's and Parkinson's. By shielding neurons from oxidative damage, C60 could help maintain cognitive function and prevent early nerve death.

Cancer Combatant: The molecule's antioxidant properties might extend to cancer prevention, protecting cells from mutations and damage that could lead to cancer.

Cardiovascular and Metabolic Marvel: C60 shows promise in preventing heart disease and diabetes by reducing oxidative stress and inflammation, supporting cardiovascular health, and stabilizing metabolic processes.

Arthritis Ally: Osteoarthritis sufferers might find relief in C60's ability to reduce inflammation and joint damage, potentially alleviating some of the pain and stiffness associated with the condition.

Buzz Around the Bucky Ball

C60 is a thrilling frontier in science and health. Its potential benefits are still being explored, but the initial findings are promising. From extending lifespan and protecting against diseases to reducing inflammation and boosting mitochondrial function, C60 is a fascinating molecule that could have a profound impact on our health and longevity.

In a nutshell, C60 is like the best-kept secret of the carbon world, and its effects on mitochondrial health, aging, and inflammation make it a star player in the quest for optimal wellness. As research continues, we might just find that this soccer-ball-shaped molecule has a lot more tricks up its sleeve.

6.2.8. Vitamin D

Vitamin D is more than just a bone buddy! Sure, it helps with calcium absorption for strong bones, but it's also your body's secret weapon for so many other things.

Vitamin D has receptors all over your body, making it a major player in immune health. It boosts antimicrobial peptides, manages your B and T-cells (the immune system's soldiers), and even helps fight off infections. Vitamin D is a known epigenetic regulator, meaning it influences which genes get turned on or off. This includes slowing down cancer cell growth and keeping inflammation in check. Plus, it's a mood booster and anti-aging superstar! How? By regulating DNA methylation, reducing oxidative stress, and pumping up your mitochondrial function—the powerhouses of your cells.

It doesn't stop there. Vitamin D activates AMPK, the enzyme that regulates your cellular energy by balancing your AMP and ATP levels (think energy production). This activation helps your body burn fat, improves glucose uptake, and boosts autophagy—your body's natural detox process that gets rid of old, damaged cells.

Want to maximize your Vitamin D? Take 5,000 to 10,000 IU per day and pair it with vitamin K2 and magnesium, both of which are needed to activate vitamin D in your body. It's easy to test your levels—just make sure they're around 40 mg/ml or 100 nmol/ml, and you're good to go!

6.3. Breathwork - The Power of Proper Breathing and CO_2 Tolerance

Most of us don't give a second thought to how we breathe, but did you know that how you inhale and exhale plays a key role in your overall health, performance, and even how much energy your cells produce?

Proper breathing isn't just about getting enough oxygen; it's about balancing the gases in your system, particularly oxygen and carbon dioxide (CO_2). Understanding the art of breathwork and improving your CO_2 tolerance can transform how your body functions at a cellular level, boosting everything from mental clarity to physical endurance.

6.3.1. The Art of Proper Breathing

Let's face it—most of us are shallow breathers. We sit slumped over computers, mindlessly breathing through our mouths, barely using our lungs to their full capacity. This type of breathing only scratches the surface, depriving our body of the benefits that come from deep, intentional breathwork. So, how do we fix this?

Proper breathing is all about diaphragmatic breathing—using your diaphragm, the muscle located just below your lungs. When you breathe deeply and correctly, your diaphragm contracts and moves downward, allowing your lungs to expand and fill with air. This simple act of deep breathing can enhance oxygen delivery to your cells and remove waste products like CO_2 more efficiently.

Here's a quick guide to start breathing properly:

1. **Inhale Slowly Through Your Nose:** Take a deep breath for about 4-6 counts, letting your belly rise as your diaphragm pulls air deep into your lungs.

2. **Exhale Slowly Through Your Nose:** Exhale for about 6-8 counts, making sure the breath is slow and controlled. Focus on squeezing out all the air and letting your belly fall naturally.
3. **Breathe with Rhythm:** Aim for about 5-6 breaths per minute, which is slower than the average person's typical 16-20 breaths per minute. This optimizes the oxygen-CO_2 exchange and allows your body to function more efficiently.

I highly encourage you to dive into daily breathwork! The absolute best app to get started with is *The Source*—a platform featuring the world's top breathwork masters!

6.3.2. The Role of CO_2 Tolerance

When we talk about breathing, oxygen always steals the spotlight, but CO_2 is just as important, if not more so. Most people think of carbon dioxide as a waste gas that we need to get rid of, but it's crucial for delivering oxygen to your cells. CO_2 tolerance is all about your body's ability to handle and regulate carbon dioxide levels without triggering a stress response (like panting or feeling anxious).

Here's how it works: When you breathe in oxygen, it binds to hemoglobin in your red blood cells. But for that oxygen to be released into your tissues and cells, you need a sufficient level of CO_2 in your bloodstream. If you exhale too quickly or shallow-breathe, you blow off too much CO_2, reducing the efficiency of oxygen delivery to your cells. This is known as the **Bohr Effect**, where a lower concentration of CO_2 reduces oxygen release from hemoglobin.

Building CO_2 tolerance helps your body handle higher levels of carbon dioxide without triggering breathlessness. With improved tolerance, your body becomes more efficient at oxygen delivery, boosting cellular energy production, improving endurance, and reducing fatigue. Athletes, for example, often use breathwork to train CO_2 tolerance and enhance their stamina and performance.

6.3.3. How to Improve CO_2 Tolerance

There are several breathwork techniques that can help you improve your CO_2 tolerance, leading to better oxygen utilization, improved cellular function, and enhanced physical and mental performance.

Controlled Breath Holds: This technique involves holding your breath after an exhale, which helps to gradually increase

CO_2 levels in your bloodstream. Here's how to do it:

- ✓ Inhale through your nose for 4 counts, then exhale slowly for 6 counts.
- ✓ After exhaling, hold your breath for as long as is comfortable without straining.
- ✓ Repeat this 4-5 times, gradually increasing your breath-hold time over the course of weeks.

Box Breathing: This is a calming breathwork technique that helps you build CO_2 tolerance while reducing stress:

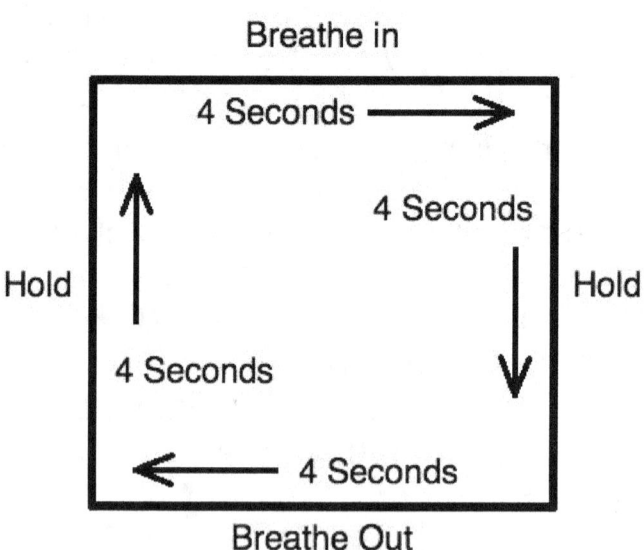

- ✓ Inhale through your nose for 4 counts.
- ✓ Hold your breath for 4 counts.
- ✓ Exhale through your nose for 4 counts.
- ✓ Hold your breath again for 4 counts before repeating the cycle.

Nasal Breathing: Simply switching from mouth breathing to nasal breathing during exercise or daily activities can help build CO_2 tolerance over time. Breathing through the nose slows down your breath and helps maintain higher CO_2 levels, ensuring better oxygen exchange.

6.3.4. Breathwork and Cellular Energy

Breathing deeply and properly does more than just calm your mind—it directly affects your body's ability to generate energy at the cellular level. When you optimize your breathing, you also improve how your mitochondria (the energy powerhouses of your cells) function. Mitochondria rely on oxygen to produce ATP (adenosine triphosphate), the molecule that powers every cell in your body. If your oxygen delivery is inefficient, your mitochondria can't produce ATP as effectively, leading to fatigue, reduced mental clarity, and poor physical performance.

Breathwork improves cellular oxygenation, helps to clear out metabolic waste like lactic acid, and enhances the body's ability to utilize oxygen for ATP production. In essence, proper breathwork supports your cells in becoming more energy-efficient, which can translate to better endurance, quicker recovery, and a boost in overall vitality.

6.3.5. The Benefits of Breathwork for Mind and Body

Beyond CO_2 tolerance and cellular energy, breathwork has a cascade of benefits:

- ✓ **Reduced Stress and Anxiety:** Controlled breathing activates the parasympathetic nervous system, reducing the "fight or flight" response and promoting relaxation.
- ✓ **Improved Focus and Mental Clarity:** By increasing oxygen flow to the brain, breathwork enhances concentration and cognitive function.
- ✓ **Enhanced Physical Performance:** Athletes use breathwork to boost endurance, improve recovery, and increase oxygen efficiency.
- ✓ **Boosted Immune Function:** Proper breathing promotes better circulation, which supports the immune system in fighting infections and disease.

Breathwork is one of the simplest, yet most powerful tools you can use to optimize your health, performance, and cellular energy. By improving your CO_2 tolerance and practicing proper breathing techniques, you can enhance how efficiently your body uses oxygen, reduce stress, and boost your overall well-being. The beauty of breathwork is that it's accessible to everyone—whether you're a high-performing athlete or just looking to improve your daily health, breathwork offers an effective way to unlock the full potential of your mind and body.

6.3.6. Breathwork and H_2 inhalation

Breathwork can amplify the benefits of molecular hydrogen (H_2) inhalation by improving oxygen and blood flow, which aids in the distribution of hydrogen throughout the body. When combined with proper breathwork, inhaling molecular hydrogen may enhance cellular absorption and efficiency.

By increasing nitric oxide production through nasal breathing, you open blood vessels and improve circulation, making it easier for hydrogen to reach tissues, muscles, and cells. This synergy can lead to faster reduction of oxidative stress, better energy production in the mitochondria, and a boost to recovery and performance, amplifying H_2's antioxidant and anti-inflammatory effects.

6.4. Skin beautification and H_2

The health and appearance of our skin are closely linked to longevity, as skin serves as both a protective barrier and a reflection of the aging process.

As we age, factors like oxidative stress, inflammation, and reduced collagen production cause visible signs of aging such as wrinkles, fine lines, and loss of elasticity. However, maintaining healthy skin can support overall longevity by safeguarding the body from environmental damage, infections, and UV radiation, all of which contribute to cellular aging.

Proper skin care, hydration, and antioxidant protection can slow down the visible signs of aging, contributing to a more youthful appearance that reflects internal health and vitality.

Thus, the condition of our skin can be a key marker of both how we age externally and how well we maintain our health over time.

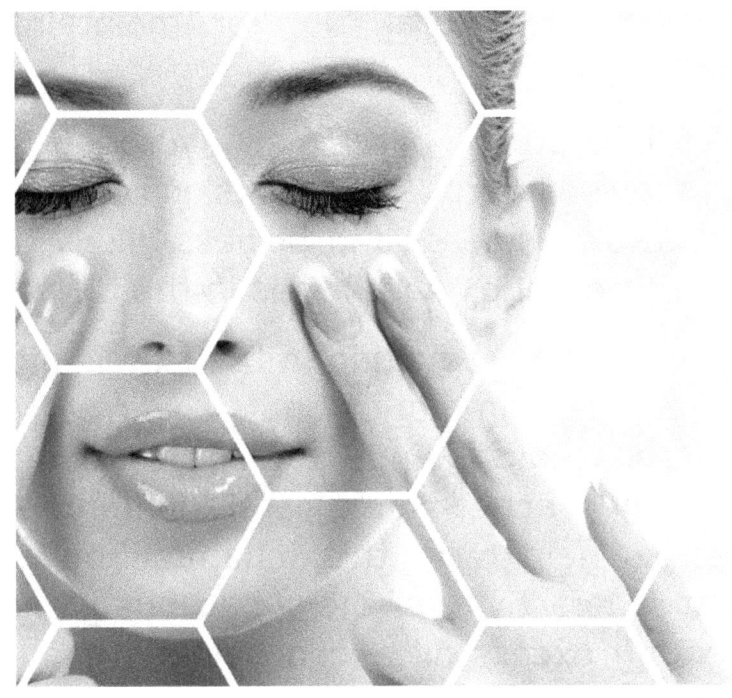

Molecular hydrogen (H$_2$) has shown promising benefits for skin health due to its powerful antioxidant and anti-inflammatory properties. By neutralizing harmful reactive oxygen species (ROS) that contribute to oxidative stress, H$_2$ helps protect skin cells from damage that can lead to premature aging, wrinkles, and dullness. Additionally, H$_2$ reduces inflammation in the skin, soothing conditions like redness, irritation, and sensitivity. Its ability to support collagen production and improve skin hydration further enhances skin elasticity and smoothness, making H_2 a natural ally for maintaining youthful, healthy skin.

In one study, bathing in hydrogen-rich water showed improvements in skin issues like wrinkles, blotchiness, and oiliness, likely due to enhanced antioxidant levels in the blood.

Excess oil production in the skin is often triggered by inflammation and an overreaction of the sebaceous glands, leading to clogged pores and acne. H_2's anti-inflammatory properties help calm this inflammation and regulate the activity of the sebaceous glands, preventing excess oil and promoting a more balanced complexion.

For dry skin, H_2 supports skin hydration by enhancing the skin's barrier function, which is crucial for retaining moisture. By neutralizing reactive oxygen species (ROS), H_2 reduces oxidative damage to the skin's lipid barrier, allowing it to better lock in moisture. This protective effect helps prevent water loss and improves overall hydration. Through its proven antioxidant and anti-inflammatory mechanisms, H_2 works to restore the skin's natural equilibrium, making it suitable for both oily and dry skin types.

Molecular hydrogen (H_2) also promotes the regeneration of epithelial skin cells by reducing oxidative stress and inflammation. By neutralizing harmful reactive oxygen species (ROS), H_2 creates an ideal environment for skin cells to heal and regenerate, accelerating repair and improving skin health. This helps maintain a strong, youthful skin barrier and supports faster recovery from damage. Additionally, H_2 enhances cellular signaling pathways involved in autophagy, where damaged components are removed, allowing for more efficient regeneration of epithelial skin cells and overall skin rejuvenation.

How Molecular Hydrogen Enhances Skin Health:

6.4.1. Reduction of Oxidative Stress

Skin aging is often accelerated by oxidative stress caused by environmental factors (such as UV radiation and pollution) and internal factors (like metabolic processes). H_2 selectively neutralizes reactive oxygen species (ROS), particularly the hydroxyl radical (•OH), which can damage skin cells and collagen.

By reducing oxidative stress, H_2 can help protect skin cells from damage, potentially reducing the appearance of wrinkles and improving skin texture and elasticity.

6.4.2. Mitigation of Inflammation

Chronic or systemic inflammation contributes to skin aging and the formation of wrinkles. H_2 has been shown to reduce the production of pro-inflammatory cytokines (e.g., TNF-α, IL-6, IL-1β) and promote anti-inflammatory cytokines (e.g., IL-10).

This anti-inflammatory effect can help reduce redness, irritation, and inflammation in the skin, contributing to a more youthful and even complexion.

6.4.3. Support of Collagen Production

Maintenance of Skin Elasticity:

Collagen is a crucial protein for maintaining skin elasticity and firmness. Oxidative stress and inflammation can degrade collagen, leading to the formation of wrinkles. By reducing oxidative damage and inflammation, H_2 may help preserve collagen levels and support the integrity of the skin matrix.

Some studies suggest that antioxidants can support collagen synthesis and prevent its breakdown, which could be beneficial for reducing wrinkles and improving skin appearance.

6.4.4. Enhancement of Skin Hydration

Improvement of Skin Barrier Function:

H_2 may help improve skin hydration by supporting the skin barrier function. A healthy skin barrier is essential for maintaining moisture and preventing dryness, which can contribute to the appearance of fine lines and wrinkles.

By promoting a healthier skin barrier, H_2 could help maintain skin hydration and reduce the visibility of wrinkles.

6.4.5. Potential for Skin Rejuvenation

Cellular Repair and Regeneration:

H_2's effects on reducing oxidative stress and inflammation can support cellular repair and regeneration processes. This can be beneficial for skin rejuvenation and the repair of damaged skin cells.

Improved cellular health and repair mechanisms can contribute to a more youthful appearance and reduced signs of aging.

6.4.6. Topical and Systemic Applications

H_2 can be administered through hydrogen-rich water, inhalation, or topical products and mists. While topical application of hydrogen-rich solutions or creams and mists provide local benefits, the use of hydrogen-rich water may offer systemic benefits that reflect on the skin's appearance.

In summary, molecular hydrogen holds potential for enhancing skin health and beauty due to its antioxidant and anti-inflammatory properties. By reducing oxidative stress and inflammation, H_2 may help prevent and reduce the appearance of wrinkles, support collagen production, and improve skin hydration. While preliminary evidence is promising, further research is needed to fully understand the benefits of H_2 for skin health and to determine the most effective methods of application for achieving these effects.

CHAPTER 7

THE NEXT FRONTIER IN ATHLETIC EXCELLENCE

Winning with H₂

Ready to transform your athletic performance and recovery? Enter molecular hydrogen (H_2), the unassuming yet powerful ally that might just redefine your fitness game. Imagine H_2 as your secret weapon, working behind the scenes to boost endurance, speed up recovery, and keep you feeling on top of your game. Here's the deep dive into how this tiny molecule delivers big results:

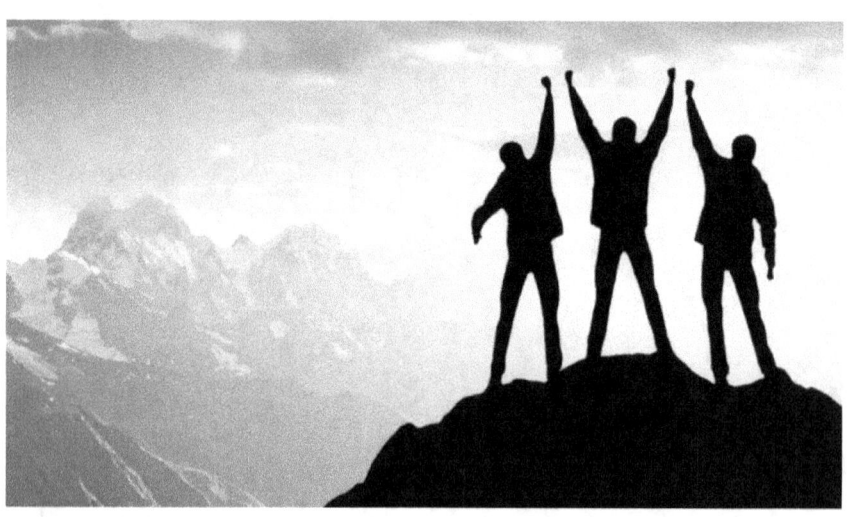

7.1. Supercharged Recovery - The Antioxidant Advantage

<u>Oxidative Stress Be Gone:</u> When you push your limits during exercise, your body produces reactive oxygen species (ROS) that can wreak havoc on your cells. These ROS, including the notorious hydroxyl radicals (•OH), are like tiny wrecking balls that cause cellular damage. H_2 steps in as a selective antioxidant, targeting these harmful radicals while leaving beneficial ROS that help with cellular signaling intact. This targeted approach helps protect your muscle cells from oxidative damage, reducing fatigue and improving your overall performance.

7.2. Inflammation Eraser - Soothe Those Sore Muscles

After a tough workout, your muscles can feel like they've been through a blender due to inflammation. H_2 combats this by reducing the production of pro-inflammatory cytokines, such as TNF-α, IL-6, and IL-1β, which contribute to muscle soreness and inflammation. At the same time, it promotes anti-inflammatory cytokines like IL-10, which helps calm things down. This dual action can result in less soreness, quicker recovery, and improved exercise performance.

7.3. Muscle Recovery Boost - Bounce Back Faster

Speedy Recovery: Intense exercise often leaves your muscles feeling damaged and sore, a phenomenon known as delayed-onset muscle soreness (DOMS). The antioxidant and anti-inflammatory properties of H_2 can help reduce this muscle damage and speed up the recovery process. Studies have shown that hydrogen-rich water or inhalation can lower markers of muscle damage and enhance recovery times, meaning you'll be back in action sooner.

7.4. Performance Power-Up - Go Further, Faster

Endurance and Strength: Athletes who incorporate hydrogen-rich water and/or inhalation into their regimen often report improved endurance and strength. Research suggests that H_2 can enhance exercise performance by boosting your stamina and reducing the perception of effort during high-intensity workouts. This means you can push harder, go longer, and recover more efficiently.

Enhanced Oxygen Utilization: H_2 may also improve how efficiently your body uses oxygen during exercise. Better oxygen utilization can lead to improved aerobic performance and a reduction in the feeling of exhaustion, making your workouts feel easier and more productive.

7.5. Fatigue Fighter - Keep the Energy Flowing

Beat the Fatigue: Exercise-induced fatigue is often a result of oxidative stress, inflammation, and muscle damage. H_2 helps tackle these fatigue-inducing factors by reducing oxidative stress and inflammation, ensuring that you can maintain your performance levels and keep fatigue at bay. This means you'll have more energy and stay strong throughout your workouts and daily activities.

7.6. Mitochondrial Mojo - Power Up Your Cells

Energy Production Pro: Mitochondria are the powerhouses of your cells, generating the energy you need to exercise. H_2 supports mitochondrial function by reducing oxidative damage and promoting mitochondrial biogenesis, the process by which new mitochondria are created. This support leads to improved energy production, better endurance, and a delay in fatigue onset during exercise.

Enhanced Mitochondrial Health: By protecting your mitochondria from damage and encouraging the growth of new mitochondria, H_2 helps ensure that your cells can keep up with the energy demands of intense physical activity. This results in more efficient energy use and improved overall performance.

7.7. Mental Clarity - Stay Sharp Under Pressure

Focus Factor: Intense physical activity can also impact your cognitive function, leading to decreased mental clarity and focus. H_2's neuroprotective effects can help maintain cognitive function and mental sharpness, ensuring you stay mentally alert and focused during and after exercise. Improved cognitive performance can be especially beneficial for athletes who need high levels of concentration and mental toughness.

7.8. Evidence on the Run - What the Science Says

From Lab to Gym: Animal studies have demonstrated that H_2 can enhance exercise performance, reduce oxidative stress, and improve recovery. These findings are backed by clinical trials involving human athletes, who have reported benefits such as better performance, reduced muscle soreness, and faster recovery times with hydrogen-rich water or hydrogen inhalation. While the early results are promising, more research is needed to fine-tune dosages and protocols for optimal benefits.

In essence, molecular hydrogen could be the game-changer your workouts have been waiting for. By reducing oxidative stress, fighting that inflammation, supporting mitochondrial health, and enhancing mental clarity, H_2 might just be the key to unlocking your full athletic potential. Dive into this powerhouse molecule and experience a new level of performance and recovery!

CHAPTER 8

NAVIGATING HYDROGEN PRODUCTS - KEY INFO FOR SAVVY CONSUMERS

It is essential for consumers to do their due diligence before making a purchase, especially when it comes to health and wellness products. The market is filled with a wide range of products, some of which make bold claims that may not be backed by solid evidence.

By thoroughly researching products, understanding the ingredients or technologies involved, and comparing various options, consumers can ensure that they are choosing items that align with their specific needs and preferences. This process helps avoid falling victim to misleading marketing or ineffective products, ensuring that the consumer's investment leads to the desired outcome.

Moreover, with the vast amount of consumer information now readily available online—ranging from user reviews to expert opinions and scientific studies—shoppers have the tools needed to make well-informed decisions. This information can help verify the efficacy and safety of products, ensuring that what consumers are purchasing is both credible and suitable for their individual requirements.

Below you will find my personal market research and key points to review so you can protect yourself from below par therapies and products, but also empower yourself to make choices that support your personal health and well-being goals.

I will discuss hydrogen tablets, hydrogen water bottles, hydrogen water units and hydrogen inhalation units. You may end up selecting the one that's right for you or decide to combine one or more products for convenience and best results.

Don't get confused by the numbers:

Milligrams (mg), cubic centimeters (cc), and parts per billion (ppb) are all units of measurement, but they measure different things, and their relationship depends on the specific context, usually involving the concentration of a substance in a solution or air.

Definitions:

- ✓ <u>Milligrams (mg)</u>: A unit of mass, where 1 mg = 1/1000th of a gram.
- ✓ <u>Cubic centimeters (cc)</u>: A unit of volume equivalent to milliliters (1 cc = 1 mL).
- ✓ <u>Parts per billion (ppb)</u>: A unit of concentration that measures the amount of a substance in a billion parts of the medium (typically air, water, or another solution). 1 ppb means 1 part of a substance per billion parts of the solution.

How They Relate:

To understand how milligrams (mg) and cubic centimeters (cc) relate to parts per billion (ppb), you need to look at concentration, which typically combines mass and volume. For instance, ppb is a mass per volume measurement, like mg/L (milligrams per liter), but on a much smaller scale.

Converting mg/L to ppb:

- ✓ 1 mg/L (milligram per liter) is equal to 1,000 ppb because 1 liter contains 1,000,000,000 (one billion) parts in the ppb scale.
- ✓ Therefore, to convert mg/L to ppb: ppb = mg/L × 1,000

- ✓ Example: 0.1 mg/L is equal to 100 ppb.
- ✓ Note: 1mg/L = 1000ppb = 1ppm.

Relating cc (mL) to mg and ppb:

- ✓ If you know the concentration of a substance in ppb and the volume of the solution in cc (mL), you can calculate the mass of the substance in mg.
- ✓ Formula to get mass in mg from ppb and cc: mg= (ppb×cc) \ 1,000,000
- ✓ Example: For a concentration of 100 ppb in 1 cc of solution, the mass of the substance would be: mg= (100×1) \ 1,000,000 =0.0001 mg

Conclusion:

- ✓ ppb measures concentration (mass per volume), while mg measures mass and cc measures volume.
- ✓ To relate them, you often need the concentration (e.g., mg/L or ppb) and the volume (e.g., cc) to calculate the mass of a substance in each solution or environment.

8.1. Hydrogen Tablets

For therapeutic use, solid-state hydrogen refers to hydrogen stored in solid materials, such as hydrogen-releasing tablets, which can deliver molecular hydrogen (H$_2$) when dissolved in water. These solid-state forms of hydrogen are designed to provide a controlled and convenient way to consume molecular hydrogen, especially for health and wellness purposes.

Hydrogen-Releasing Tablets:

Mechanism: Solid hydrogen tablets typically contain compounds such as magnesium, which react with water to release molecular hydrogen gas (H$_2$). Once dissolved, the water becomes hydrogen-rich and is consumed.

Advantages: These tablets are easy to use, portable, and provide a consistent dose of molecular hydrogen.

Disadvantages: (1) Metallic taste from elemental magnesium, (2) need to consume immediately since the hydrogen is unstable, (3) often not exact knowledge about cc/l or ppb.

Dosage: Typically, 1-3 tablets per day, depending on the strength and intended therapeutic effects, which can release hydrogen concentrations of 2-8 mg per tablet. I use a tablet with a dose of 12ppm = 12000 ppb = 12ml/l or 12cc/l.

Like tablets, hydrogen can also be delivered through powders or capsules that release hydrogen once ingested or dissolved in a liquid.

Most tablets sell for $40-$50 for a month supply.

8.2. Hydrogen Devices

While a simple chemical reaction releases hydrogen from tablets, hydrogen units employ other methods to produce stable molecular hydrogen. These methods are used in hydrogen bottles, home units and commercial units that produce hydrogenated water or hydrogen gas for inhalation, or both.

8.2.1. Electrolysis Magic

Electrolysis involves using an electric current to split water (H_2O) into hydrogen (H_2) and oxygen (O_2) gases. Water is placed in an electrolysis device, where electricity is passed through electrodes.

The positive electrode (anode) generates oxygen, and the negative electrode (cathode) generates hydrogen. The hydrogen is stable and can be stored and is 99.9% pure. The average concentration in hydrogen water is 1.7cc/liter.

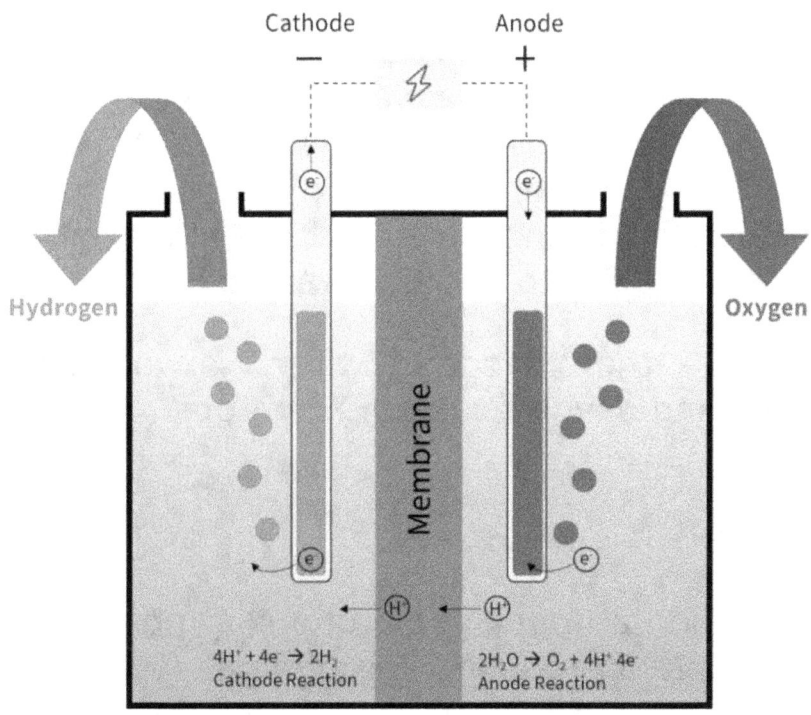

8.2.2. Proton Exchange Membranes

A Proton Exchange Membrane (PEM) is a technology used to produce therapeutic hydrogen through the electrolysis of water. This method is popular for its efficiency and ability to produce high-purity hydrogen with minimal environmental impact, especially when used for therapeutic applications like hydrogen inhalation or hydrogen-rich water.

How PEM Electrolysis Works:

PEM electrolysis uses a solid polymer electrolyte (SPE) membrane that conducts protons from the anode (positive electrode) to the cathode (negative electrode) while keeping oxygen and hydrogen gases separated. When an electric current is applied, water is split into hydrogen and oxygen.

At the anode, water is oxidized, producing oxygen gas (O_2), protons (H^+), and electrons (e^-):

$$2H_2O \rightarrow O_2 + 4H^+ + 4e^-$$

At the cathode, the protons combine with electrons to produce hydrogen gas (H_2):

$$4H^+ + 4e^- \rightarrow 2H_2$$

Pure Hydrogen Production:

The PEM allows only protons (H^+) to pass through, ensuring the separation of hydrogen and oxygen. This produces high-purity hydrogen gas without any hazardous by-products, which is ideal for medical or therapeutic use.

8.3. Hydrogen water vs. Inhalation

Hydrogen water advantages:

Ease of Use: Hydrogen water is easy to consume and easy to integrate into daily routines. It can be made at home with hydrogen water generators or purchased as pre-packaged hydrogen water.

Systemic Absorption: Once ingested, H_2 is absorbed through the digestive system and enters the bloodstream, where it may exert its antioxidant and anti-inflammatory effects throughout the body.

GI and Gut: when drinking hydrogen water, molecular hydrogen comes into direct contact with the gut. Therefore, hydrogen water may be a better delivery method when dealing with GI, digestive and gut problems.

Portable: Hydrogen water can be consumed anywhere, making it a convenient option for regular use, especially for athletes or individuals on the go.

Limitations:

Lower Concentration: The amount of H_2 that can dissolve in water is limited, ranging from 0.5 to 1.7 mg/L of hydrogen, depending on the method of infusion. So, the total dosage may be significantly lower compared to inhalation.

Short Shelf Life: Hydrogen gas dissipates from water relatively quickly, so hydrogen-rich water must be consumed shortly after production for maximum benefits.

Hydrogen Inhalation:

The inhalation method usually delivers 1-4% hydrogen mixed with air, and the gas is absorbed directly into the bloodstream through the lungs.

High Concentration: Inhalation allows for a much higher dose of molecular hydrogen compared to drinking hydrogen-rich water. The body can absorb a larger amount of hydrogen in a shorter time.

Various devices will have different flow rates. For example, some home units produce 300, 600 or 1200cc/minute while some commercial units can produce up to 3000cc/minute. The better devices have a concentration of 4-4.3% of hydrogen. This means that if, for example, we use a 600cc/minute device, we inhale 24cc of hydrogen/min or 360cc of hydrogen in just 15 minutes.

To consume 360cc of hydrogen by drinking hydrogen water at 1.7cc/liter, we would need to drink 211 liters or 62 gallons. We can get 360cc by inhalation for only 15 minutes with a 600cc/min flowrate device.

Rapid Absorption: Hydrogen inhalation offers faster and more efficient absorption, as molecular hydrogen is directly taken into the lungs and quickly diffuses into the bloodstream.

Neuroprotective Effects: Studies suggest that hydrogen inhalation may have particularly strong neuroprotective effects, making it useful for conditions like stroke, neuro-degenerative diseases, or traumatic brain injuries.

Localized Benefits: Inhalation may target organs more effectively, especially the lungs and brain, due to its direct delivery through the respiratory system.

Limitations:

Requires Equipment: Hydrogen inhalation typically requires a dedicated inhalation device, which may be less convenient than simply drinking water. However, over time this may be better investment with water being the only consumable.

Time Commitment: Inhalation sessions can last between 30 minutes to 2 hours or longer, depending on the therapeutic goal, which may not be as practical for some users.

Portability: While there are portable hydrogen inhalation devices, they are less convenient than hydrogen water for use on the go.

Comparison Summary:

Speed of Effect: Inhalation may deliver quicker results due to direct entry into the bloodstream. Hydrogen water provides more gradual benefits as hydrogen needs to be absorbed through the digestive system.

Effectiveness: Inhalation may be more effective for acute conditions due to higher hydrogen levels. Hydrogen-rich water is great for general health maintenance and GI issues, where direct contact with the gut is beneficial.

Consider Dual Therapy:

Combining both inhalation and hydrogen water might be your best bet. After all, we drink water daily, so why not make it hydrogen-rich? Dual therapy can optimize your health and combat disease more effectively. You may consider devices designed for both inhalation and hydrogen water or two separate units based on your needs and desires.

Hydrogen water versus inhalation:

Aspect	H_2 water	H_2 inhalation
concentration	Lower (0,5-1.7 ml/l)	Higher (1-4% H_2 gas)
absorption speed	Slower (digestive system)	Faster (lungs into blood)
benefits	General wellness, antioxidant, anti-inflammatory	Neuro-protection, faster recovery, higher dosage
convenience	Easy to consume, portable	Requires inhalation device, less portable
use	Daily wellness, skin health, metabolism	Targeted therapy for brain, lungs, faster results
time	Quick (just drinking)	Longer sessions (30 min to 2+ hours)

8.4. Not All Devices Are Created Equally

When it comes to hydrogen devices, quality matters! Here's what you need to know:

8.4.1. Hydrogen Catalysts

A catalyst is a substance that increases the rate of a chemical reaction without itself undergoing any permanent chemical change.

To this extent, I would like to emphasize the importance of using only white gold and platinum as hydrogen catalysts. It's crucial to caution against using lye (industrial salt), citric acid, and sodium hydroxide. So be aware of cheap, poorly made devices, especially those from less reputable manufacturers. Often inferior materials are used that can oxidize quickly, unlike platinum and white gold. Look for devices with a run-time of at least 5 hours and up to 24 hours and a guarantee of over 5,000 hours to ensure quality.

8.4.2. Quality Considerations

Especially for chronic and degenerative diseases, it's important to use the highest quality equipment.

If you are a health care practitioner and considering a commercial unit, it's imperative you purchase a high-end device with the highest quality standards.

But in general, look for the following:

- ✓ Look for systems that guarantee pure molecular hydrogen inhalation.
- ✓ High-end units can run continuously, allowing clients to sleep with the cannula attached (longer run times).
- ✓ High-end units require a larger tank with sterile/distilled water.
- ✓ Hydrogen analysis: The best devices come with sensors to monitor hydrogen production, purity, and more. They should include automatic alerts and shut-off features if water quality is inadequate.
- ✓ High-end systems have introduced additional features such as:
    - o Eye goggles for macular degeneration, floaters, eye hydration, and brain fog.
    - o Hydrogen boots for diabetic wound care.
    - o Other add-ons that extend the system's benefits.
- ✓ <u>Hydrogen-Oxygen Mix:</u> Some units combine hydrogen with oxygen (oxyhydrogen gas or brown gas). In

theory, the combined presence of hydrogen and oxygen could offer unique therapeutic properties. For instance, oxygen could support additional healing processes in combination with hydrogen's effects.

8.4.3. Cost Considerations

<u>Hydrogen Tablets</u> are the most affordable ($40-$50/month) and portable but require continuous purchase.

<u>Hydrogen Water bottles</u> offer convenience and deliver 1.2-4.5 ppm of H_2. They run between $100-$300, no consumables needed, just water.

<u>Home Hydrogen Water Generators</u> provide the most cost-effective solution for long-term, daily hydrogen water consumption. They range from $1000-$5000. Filters are consumables.

<u>Hydrogen Inhalation Devices</u> deliver higher concentrations of hydrogen, ideal for those with specific health conditions, but come with a higher upfront cost. The cost increases with the flowrate and run-time. Home units with a flow rate of 300cc/l to 1800cc/l range from $3000-$9000 and commercial units with flow rates of 2000 to 3000cc/l range from $9000-

$20000. Commercial devices are suited for clinics and wellness centers.

Some devices offer both hydrogen-rich water and inhalation.

Some companies offer payment plans or rentals to make it easier to access high-quality devices.

Investing in a quality device ensures you get the most out of your hydrogen therapy, whether you're enhancing your daily health or targeting specific conditions.

To discuss the best devices on the market today or simply chat with me about molecular hydrogen and how it can work for you, feel free to schedule a free 20-min. consultation on my website. You can also visit my webpage on molecular hydrogen to review the companies selling these devices and the discounts offered:

8.5. Safety and Dosing – The Lowdown

The therapeutic dosage of molecular hydrogen (H_2) can vary depending on the method of delivery, the condition being treated, and individual factors. However, research suggests general guidelines for therapeutic use:

Hydrogen-Rich Water (Drinking)

- ✓ Concentration: Therapeutic levels of hydrogen in water typically range from 0.5 to 1.7 mg/L (milligrams per liter), also expressed as 0.5 to 1.7 ppm (parts per million).
- ✓ Dosage: Studies often use doses of about 1-3 liters per day of hydrogen-rich water. Drinking 500 mL to 1 liter of hydrogen-rich water twice a day is a common therapeutic regimen.
- ✓ Timing: It's usually recommended to consume hydrogen-rich water on an empty stomach for better absorption, as hydrogen can dissipate in the presence of food and other substances.

Hydrogen Inhalation (Gas)

- ✓ Concentration: Inhaling 1-4% hydrogen gas mixed with air is considered safe and therapeutically effective.

- ✓ Dosage: Inhalation sessions typically last 30 minutes to 2 hours depending on the condition being treated. Regular inhalation (daily or a few times a week) can be used for chronic conditions or for recovery, such as after exercise or in medical treatments.
- ✓ Delivery Devices: Hydrogen inhalation devices deliver controlled amounts of hydrogen gas, ensuring safe and consistent dosages.

Hydrogen Tablets or Capsules

- ✓ Dosage: Hydrogen tablets that dissolve in water typically release 2-8 mg of hydrogen per tablet. Some formulations are designed to release higher concentrations in smaller volumes of water, making it convenient for therapeutic use.
- ✓ Frequency: Most recommendations suggest taking 1-3 tablets per day, depending on the tablet's strength and the specific health goals.

Bathing or Topical Applications

- ✓ Concentration: When used in hydrogen baths, concentrations of around 1-4 ppm can provide therapeutic benefits for skin and muscle recovery.

- ✓ **Duration:** Bathing for 15-30 minutes in hydrogen-infused water allows for absorption through the skin, which can be useful for localized pain, inflammation, and skin conditions.

General Guidelines:

- ✓ **Daily Intake:** For preventive health and general wellness, 1-2 mg of molecular hydrogen per day is often sufficient, which can be achieved through drinking hydrogen-rich water or using other delivery methods.
- ✓ **Higher Doses:** For specific therapeutic purposes or chronic conditions (e.g., neurodegenerative diseases, metabolic disorders), higher doses of 4-8 mg/day may be recommended based on research studies.

Dosing Guidelines (Not Medical Advice!):

For cancer and chronic diseases, you might want to aim for a flow rate of 600-3000cc/min, for 2-8 hours a day.

Prevention, longevity, and athletic performance? Try 300-900cc/min for 1-2 hours a day, or 3-4 times a week. If better sleep is your goal, a 1-hour session near bedtime works wonders.

For <u>acute pain or other symptoms</u>, crank it up to the highest available flow rate for 2 hours, repeating twice a day until symptoms subside.

When you drink hydrogenated water at 1.7cc/liter, you can't overdo it either. While drinking ample water is key to good health, forcing excess water down your throat can be dangerous.

When you drink hydrogenated water or inhale hydrogen gas, the H_2 is carried by your blood plasma straight to your cells. The cool part? Hydrogen reaches its saturation point in your blood at 1.8-2.2 cc/liter, and any excess is simply exhaled. So, you can't really "overdose" on hydrogen—your body knows exactly what to do with the extra!

It's important to note that molecular hydrogen is considered safe even at higher concentrations, as it is a naturally occurring molecule in the body with no known toxic effects. However, for specific medical conditions, it's always advisable to consult with a healthcare provider familiar with hydrogen therapy.

In addition, quality devices used for hydrogen inhalation deliver 99.99% pure molecular hydrogen at a concentration of

4.3% or less, making it safe and non-flammable.

The FDA has given hydrogen gas the Generally Recognized as Safe (GRAS) stamp of approval for certain uses, particularly in food and beverages like hydrogen-infused water.

However, this GRAS status doesn't extend to therapeutic or medical applications just yet—those are still being studied. So, while hydrogen's health benefits, from combating oxidative stress to improving immune function, are being explored, it hasn't crossed the FDA's finish line as an official medical treatment.

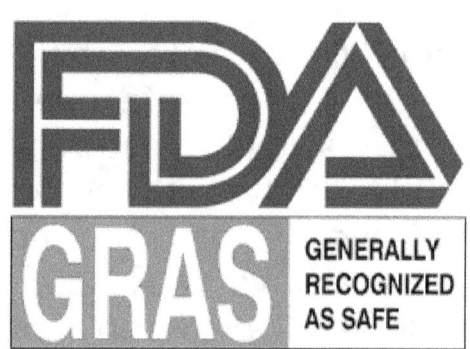

Remember, these are general guidelines, not medical advice. Personalization is key!

MOLECULAR HYDOGEN – NEW HOPE

REFERENCES – SCIENTIFIC LITERATURE

For easy access, you may also find all references here:

Allergies

https://pubmed.ncbi.nlm.nih.gov/19766097/

Molecular hydrogen suppresses FcepsilonRI-mediated signal transduction and prevents degranulation of mast cells.

Alzheimer's

https://www.ncbi.nlm.nih.gov/pmc/articles/PMC9224395/

Molecular Hydrogen Neuroprotection in Post-Ischemic Neurodegeneration in the Form of Alzheimer's Disease Proteinopathy:

Underlying Mechanisms and Potential for Clinical Implementation—Fantasy or Reality?

Anti-inflammatory / Antioxidant properties

https://pubmed.ncbi.nlm.nih.gov/23031079/ Consumption of water containing a high concentration of molecular hydrogen reduces oxidative stress and disease activity in patients with rheumatoid arthritis: an open-label pilot study

https://www.ncbi.nlm.nih.gov/pmc/articles/PMC3788323/ Molecular hydrogen: new antioxidant and anti-inflammatory therapy for rheumatoid arthritis and related diseases

https://pubmed.ncbi.nlm.nih.gov/11510417/ Anti-inflammatory properties of molecular hydrogen: investigation on parasite-induced liver inflammation.

https://www.ncbi.nlm.nih.gov/pmc/articles/PMC7871940/
Hydrogen-rich water suppresses the reduction in blood total antioxidant capacity induced by 3 consecutive days of severe exercise in physically active males

https://www.ncbi.nlm.nih.gov/pmc/articles/PMC7376192/
Hydrogen-rich water reduces inflammatory responses and prevents apoptosis of

peripheral blood cells in healthy adults: a randomized, double-blind, controlled trial

https://www.ncbi.nlm.nih.gov/pmc/articles/PMC6988658/
Application of Molecular Hydrogen as a Novel Antioxidant in Sports Science

https://www.ncbi.nlm.nih.gov/pmc/articles/PMC6096066/
Anti-inflammatory and antitumor action of hydrogen via reactive oxygen species

https://pubmed.ncbi.nlm.nih.gov/30243702/
Molecular hydrogen reduces acute exercise-induced inflammatory and oxidative stress status

https://www.ncbi.nlm.nih.gov/pmc/articles/PMC10045005/
Molecular Hydrogen: From Molecular Effects to Stem Cells Management and Tissue Regeneration

https://www.ncbi.nlm.nih.gov/pmc/articles/PMC5095341/
(2016) Molecular hydrogen decelerates rheumatoid arthritis progression through inhibition of oxidative stress

https://www.sciencedirect.com/science/article/pii/S1567576914002124?ref=pdf_download
(2014) Therapeutic efficacy of infused

molecular hydrogen in saline on rheumatoid arthritis: A randomized, double-blind, placebo-controlled pilot study

https://www.ncbi.nlm.nih.gov/pmc/articles/PMC3563451/
(2012) Consumption of water containing a high concentration of molecular hydrogen reduces oxidative stress and disease activity in patients with rheumatoid arthritis: an open-label pilot study

https://www.spandidos-publications.com/10.3892/etm.2018.6880
(2018) Beneficial Effects of Hydrogen Gas Inhalation on a Murine Model of Allergic Rhinitis

Antioxidant & Brain Protection

https://pubmed.ncbi.nlm.nih.gov/17486089/
Hydrogen acts as a therapeutic antioxidant by selectively reducing cytotoxic oxygen radicals

https://www.ncbi.nlm.nih.gov/pmc/articles/PMC3694409/Safety of intravenous administration of hydrogen-enriched fluid in patients with acute cerebral ischemia: initial clinical studies

https://www.ncbi.nlm.nih.gov/pmc/articles/PMC4865993/A randomized double-blind multi-center trial of hydrogen water for

Parkinson's disease: protocol and baseline characteristics

https://www.ncbi.nlm.nih.gov/pmc/articles/PMC10057981/ Therapeutic Inhalation of Hydrogen Gas for Alzheimer's Disease Patients and Subsequent Long-Term Follow-Up as a Disease-Modifying Treatment: An Open Label Pilot Study

https://pubmed.ncbi.nlm.nih.gov/28669654/ Hydrogen Gas Inhalation Treatment in Acute Cerebral Infarction: A Randomized Controlled Clinical Study on Safety and Neuroprotection

https://www.ncbi.nlm.nih.gov/pmc/articles/PMC6664236/

Effects of Molecular Hydrogen on Methamphetamine-Induced Neurotoxicity and Spatial Memory Impairment

https://www.ncbi.nlm.nih.gov/pmc/articles/PMC6087877/ Hydrogen-Rich Water Ameliorates Autistic-Like Behavioral Abnormalities in Valproic Acid-Treated Adolescent Mice Offspring

Asthma-Allergic Inflammation

https://www.nature.com/articles/s41598-020-58999-0
Hydrogen Attenuates Allergic Inflammation by Reversing Energy Metabolic Pathway

Switch Scientific

https://www.sciencedirect.com/science/article/abs/pii/S1567576918313638
Hydrogen gas inhalation enhances alveolar macrophage phagocytosis in an ovalbumin-induced asthma model

Athletic & Muscle Performance

https://www.ncbi.nlm.nih.gov/pmc/articles/PMC3395574/
Pilot study: Effects of drinking hydrogen-rich water on muscle fatigue caused by acute exercise in elite athletes

https://pubmed.ncbi.nlm.nih.gov/28474871/
Effects of hydrogen rich water on prolonged intermittent exercise

https://pubmed.ncbi.nlm.nih.gov/25295663/
Effectiveness of oral and topical hydrogen for sports-related soft tissue injuries

https://www.ncbi.nlm.nih.gov/pmc/articles/PMC6837388/
Molecular hydrogen alleviates motor deficits and muscle degeneration in mdx mice

Bioavailability & Inhalation

https://www.ncbi.nlm.nih.gov/pmc/articles/PMC5731988/
Molecular hydrogen: a preventive and

therapeutic medical gas for various diseases

https://pubmed.ncbi.nlm.nih.gov/21621588/
Molecular hydrogen is a novel antioxidant to efficiently reduce oxidative stress with potential for the improvement of mitochondrial diseases

https://pubmed.ncbi.nlm.nih.gov/17486089/
Hydrogen acts as a therapeutic antioxidant by selectively reducing cytotoxic oxygen radicals

https://pubmed.ncbi.nlm.nih.gov/18563058/
Consumption of molecular hydrogen prevents the stress-induced impairments in hippocampus-dependent learning tasks during chronic physical restraint in mice

https://pubmed.ncbi.nlm.nih.gov/24769081/
Molecular hydrogen as a preventive and therapeutic medical gas: initiation, development and potential of hydrogen medicine

https://pubmed.ncbi.nlm.nih.gov/28669654/
Hydrogen Gas Inhalation Treatment in Acute Cerebral Infarction: A Randomized Controlled Clinical Study on Safety and Neuroprotection

Cancer

https://www.mdpi.com/1422-0067/22/16/8724

Molecular Hydrogen as a Novel Antitumor Agent: Possible Mechanisms Underlying Gene Expression

https://www.sciencedirect.com/science/article/pii/S0163725814000941?via%3Dihub
Molecular hydrogen as a preventive and therapeutic medical gas: initiation, development and potential of hydrogen medicine

https://www.mdpi.com/2571-8797/2/4/33
Hydrogen Is Promising for Medical Applications

https://www.ncbi.nlm.nih.gov/pmc/articles/PMC8123813/
Molecular Hydrogen as a Potential Clinically Applicable Radioprotective Agent

https://www.ncbi.nlm.nih.gov/pmc/articles/PMC3805896/
Hydrogen as a New Class of Radioprotective Agent

https://www.ncbi.nlm.nih.gov/pmc/articles/PMC7189362/
Hydrogen gas represses the progression of lung cancer via down-regulating CD47

https://www.ncbi.nlm.nih.gov/pmc/articles/PMC7885710/
Hydrogen therapy can be used to control tumor progression and alleviate the adverse

events of medications in patients with advanced non-small cell lung cancer

https://www.ncbi.nlm.nih.gov/pmc/articles/PMC8092147/
Two weeks of hydrogen inhalation can significantly reverse adaptive and innate immune system senescence patients with advanced non-small cell lung cancer: a self-controlled study

https://www.ncbi.nlm.nih.gov/pmc/articles/PMC7448556/
Suppression of autophagy facilitates hydrogen gas-mediated lung cancer cell apoptosis

https://www.ncbi.nlm.nih.gov/pmc/articles/PMC6691140/
Hydrogen Gas in Cancer Treatment

https://pdfs.semanticscholar.org/cf12/d0164bf19ab13b57594757554c3b52a4df04.pdf
Neutral pH Hydrogen-Enriched Electrolyzed Water Achieves Tumor-Preferential Clonal Growth Inhibition Over Normal Cells and Tumor Invasion Inhibition Concurrently With Intracellular Oxidant Repression

https://pubmed.ncbi.nlm.nih.gov/19783965/
Platinum nanocolloid-supplemented hydrogendissolved water inhibits growth of human tongue carcinoma cells preferentially

over normal cells

https://pubmed.ncbi.nlm.nih.gov/21042740/
Antitumor effects of nano-bubble hydrogen-dissolved water are enhanced by coexistent platinum colloid and the combined hyperthermia with apoptosis-like cell death

https://www.tandfonline.com/doi/full/10.3109/10715762.2015.1131823
Transient generation of hydrogen peroxide is responsible for carcinostatic effects of hydrogen combined with platinum nanocolloid, together with increases intracellular ROS, DNA cleavages, and proportion of G2/M-phase

https://pubmed.ncbi.nlm.nih.gov/33387361/
Carcinostatic effects of alkanoyl ascorbate plus platinum nano-colloid and stabilization of the esterolytically resultant ascorbate by hydrogen

https://www.scientific.net/MSF.706-709.520
Influence of Hydrogen Discharged from Palladium Base Hydrogen Storage Alloys on Cancer Cells

https://peerj.com/articles/859/
Hydrogen–water enhances 5-fluorouracil-induced inhibition of colon cancer

https://www.sciencedirect.com/science/article/abs/pii/S0753332218308667?via%3Dihub

Hydrogen gas inhibits lung cancer progression through targeting SMC3

https://pubmed.ncbi.nlm.nih.gov/31113492/
Molecular hydrogen suppresses glioblastoma growth via inducing the glioma stem-like cell differentiation

https://pubmed.ncbi.nlm.nih.gov/31924176/
Hydrogen inhibits endometrial cancer growth via a ROS/NLRP3/caspase-1/GSDMD-mediated pyroptotic pathway

https://aasldpubs.onlinelibrary.wiley.com/doi/10.1002/hep.25782
Hydrogen-rich water prevents progression of nonalcoholic steatohepatitis and accompanying hepatocarcinogenesis in mice†

https://www.jstage.jst.go.jp/article/bpb/31/1/31_1_19/_article
Inhibitory Effect of Electrolyzed Reduced Water on Tumor Angiogenesis

https://www.spandidos-publications.com/10.3892/or.2018.6841
Hydrogen gas restores exhausted CD8+ T cells in patients with advanced colorectal cancer to improve prognosis

https://www.spandidos-publications.com/10.3892/ol.2020.12121
Hydrogen gas activates coenzyme Q10 to restore exhausted CD8+ T cells, especially

PD-1+Tim3+terminal CD8+ T cells, leading to better nivolumab outcomes in patients with lung cancer

https://pubmed.ncbi.nlm.nih.gov/31552873/
"Real world survey" of hydrogen-controlled cancer: a follow-up report of 82 advanced cancer patients

https://www.sciencedirect.com/science/article/pii/S0163725814000941?via%3Dihub
Molecular hydrogen as a preventive and therapeutic medical gas: initiation, development and potential of hydrogen medicine

https://www.mdpi.com/1422-0067/22/5/2549
Potential Therapeutic Applications of Hydrogen in Chronic Inflammatory Diseases: Possible Inhibiting Role on Mitochondrial Stress

https://www.wjgnet.com/2307-8960/full/v7/i15/2065.htm
Hydrogen gas therapy induced shrinkage of metastatic gallbladder cancer: A case report

https://www.dovepress.com/a-gallbladder-carcinoma-patient-with-pseudo-progressive-remission-afte-peer-reviewed-fulltext-article-OTT
A Gallbladder Carcinoma Patient With

Pseudo-Progressive Remission After Hydrogen Inhalation

https://www.dovepress.com/brain-metastases-completely-disappear-in-non-small-cell-lung-cancer-us-peer-reviewed-fulltext-article-OTT
Brain Metastases Completely Disappear in Non-Small Cell Lung Cancer Using Hydrogen Gas Inhalation: A Case Report

https://journals.lww.com/mgar/fulltext/2020/10020/hydrogen_therapy_can_be_used_to_control_tumor.5.aspx
Hydrogen therapy can be used to control tumor progression and alleviate the adverse events of medications in patients with advanced non-small cell lung cancer

https://www.sciencedirect.com/science/article/abs/pii/S0753332218308667?via%3Dihub
Hydrogen gas inhibits lung cancer progression through targeting SMC3

https://stemcellres.biomedcentral.com/articles/10.1186/s13287-019-1241-x
Molecular hydrogen suppresses glioblastoma growth via inducing the glioma stem-like cell differentiation

https://bmccancer.biomedcentral.com/articles/10.1186/s12885-019-6491-6
Hydrogen inhibits endometrial cancer growth

via a ROS/NLRP3/caspase-1/GSDMD-mediated pyroptotic pathway

https://www.jstage.jst.go.jp/article/bpb/31/1/31_1_19/_article
Inhibitory Effect of Electrolyzed Reduced Water on Tumor Angiogenesis

https://www.ingentaconnect.com/content/tsp/or/2008/00000017/00000006/art00002;jsessionid=5kbn5mmmbtcs1.x-ic-live-03
Neutral pH Hydrogen-Enriched Electrolyzed Water Achieves Tumor-Preferential Clonal Growth Inhibition Over Normal Cells and Tumor Invasion Inhibition Concurrently With Intracellular Oxidant Repression

https://pubmed.ncbi.nlm.nih.gov/21042740/
Antitumor effects of nano-bubble hydrogen-dissolved water are enhanced by coexistent platinum colloid and the combined hyperthermia with apoptosis-like cell death

https://www.tandfonline.com/doi/full/10.3109/10715762.2015.1131823
Transient generation of hydrogen peroxide is responsible for carcinostatic effects of hydrogen combined with platinum nanocolloid, together with increases intracellular ROS, DNA cleavages, and proportion of G2/M-phase

https://link.springer.com/article/10.1007/s13

577-020-00462-3
Carcinostatic effects of alkanoyl ascorbate plus platinum nano-colloid and stabilization of the esterolytically resultant ascorbate by hydrogen

https://www.ajol.info/index.php/tjpr/article/view/164283
Potential protective role of hydrogen against cisplatininduced side effects during chemotherapy: A mini-review of a novel hypothesis for antagonism of hydrogen

https://pubmed.ncbi.nlm.nih.gov/29142752/
Protective effect of hydrogen-rich water on liver function of colorectal cancer patients treated with mFOLFOX6 chemotherapy

https://pubmed.ncbi.nlm.nih.gov/19249288/
Hydrogen-rich saline reduces lung injury induced by intestinal ischemia/reperfusion in rats

https://pubmed.ncbi.nlm.nih.gov/18996093/
Consumption of hydrogen water prevents atherosclerosis in apolipoprotein E knockout mice

https://www.spandidos-publications.com/10.3892/or.2018.6841
Hydrogen gas restores exhausted CD8+ T cells in patients with advanced colorectal cancer to improve prognosis

https://www.researchsquare.com/article/rs-201468/v1
Investigating the Effect of Hydrogen-Rich Water on Liver Cell Injury and Liver Cancer by Regulating GP73/ TGF-β Pathway

https://www.spandidos-publications.com/10.3892/or.2021.8092
Mechanism of hydrogen on cervical cancer suppression revealed by high-throughput RNA sequencing

https://bmccancer.biomedcentral.com/articles/10.1186/s12885-019-6491-6
Hydrogen inhibits endometrial cancer growth via a ROS/NLRP3/caspase-1/GSDMD-mediated pyroptotic pathway

https://onlinelibrary.wiley.com/doi/10.1155/2022/8024452
Molecular Hydrogen Inhibits Colorectal Cancer Growth via the AKT/SCD1 Signaling Pathway

https://www.spandidos-publications.com/10.3892/or.2018.6841
Hydrogen gas restores exhausted CD8+ T cells in patients with advanced colorectal cancer to improve prognosis

https://pubmed.ncbi.nlm.nih.gov/19148645/
Molecular hydrogen alleviates nephrotoxicity induced by an anti-cancer drug cisplatin

without compromising anti-tumor activity in mice

https://pubmed.ncbi.nlm.nih.gov/20505032/
Experimental verification of protective effect of hydrogen-rich water against cisplatin-induced nephrotoxicity in rats using dynamic contrast-enhanced CT

https://pubmed.ncbi.nlm.nih.gov/22146004/
Effects of drinking hydrogen-rich water on the quality of life of patients treated with radiotherapy for liver tumors

https://pubmed.ncbi.nlm.nih.gov/32541132/
Hydrogen therapy can be used to control tumor progression and alleviate the adverse events of medications in patients with advanced non-small cell lung cancer

https://pubmed.ncbi.nlm.nih.gov/26668628/
Hydrogen-rich saline attenuates chemotherapy-induced ovarian injury via regulation of oxidative stress

https://www.nature.com/articles/nm1577
Hydrogen acts as a therapeutic antioxidant by selectively reducing cytotoxic oxygen radicals

https://www.ncbi.nlm.nih.gov/pmc/articles/PMC5666661/
Protective effect of hydrogen-rich water on liver function of colorectal cancer patients

treated with mFOLFOX6 chemotherapy

Cardiovascular disease

https://www.ncbi.nlm.nih.gov/pmc/articles/PMC6600250/
A New Approach for the Prevention and Treatment of Cardiovascular Disorders. Molecular Hydrogen Significantly Reduces the Effects of Oxidative Stress

https://www.ncbi.nlm.nih.gov/pmc/articles/PMC8353690/
Application of Molecular Hydrogen in Heart Surgery under Cardiopulmonary Bypass

https://www.ncbi.nlm.nih.gov/pmc/articles/PMC9555031/
Molecular hydrogen exposure improves functional state of red blood cells in the early postoperative period: a randomized clinical study

https://www.ncbi.nlm.nih.gov/pmc/articles/PMC10239052/
Hydrogen therapy as a potential therapeutic intervention in heart disease: from the past evidence to future application

https://pubmed.ncbi.nlm.nih.gov/25979689%20
Treatment with hydrogen molecule attenuates cardiac dysfunction in

streptozotocin-induced diabetic mice

COPD

https://www.ncbi.nlm.nih.gov/pmc/articles/PMC8120708/
Hydrogen/oxygen therapy for the treatment of an acute exacerbation of chronic obstructive pulmonary disease: results of a multicenter, randomized, double-blind, parallel group controlled trial

https://www.ncbi.nlm.nih.gov/pmc/articles/PMC7785302/
Hydrogen gas (XEN) inhalation ameliorates airway inflammation in asthma and COPD patients

https://www.ncbi.nlm.nih.gov/pmc/articles/PMC6051853/
Hydrogen gas inhalation protects against cigarette smoke-induced COPD development in mice

https://www.ncbi.nlm.nih.gov/pmc/articles/PMC3108576/
Hydrogen Therapy may be a Novel and Effective Treatment for COPD

COVID

https://www.ncbi.nlm.nih.gov/pmc/articles/PMC8569706/
(2121) Molecular Hydrogen: A Promising

Adjunctive Strategy for the Treatment of the COVID-19

https://www.ncbi.nlm.nih.gov/pmc/articles/PMC8896485/
Hydrogen-oxygen therapy alleviates clinical symptoms in twelve patients hospitalized with COVID-19

https://www.ncbi.nlm.nih.gov/pmc/articles/PMC8872486/
Molecular Hydrogen Positively Affects Physical and Respiratory Function in Acute Post-COVID-19 Patients: A New Perspective in Rehabilitation

https://www.ncbi.nlm.nih.gov/pmc/articles/PMC7330772/
Hydrogen/oxygen mixed gas inhalation improves disease severity and dyspnea in patients with Coronavirus disease 2019 in a recent multicenter, open-label clinical trial

Diabetes

https://pubmed.ncbi.nlm.nih.gov/19083400/
Supplementation of hydrogen-rich water improves lipid and glucose metabolism in patients with type 2 diabetes or impaired glucose tolerance

https://www.ncbi.nlm.nih.gov/pmc/articles/PMC3542317/
(2013) Hydrogen Improves Glycemic Control

in Type1 Diabetic Animal Model by Promoting Glucose Uptake into Skeletal Muscle

https://www.ncbi.nlm.nih.gov/pmc/articles/PMC3542317/
(2020) Hydrogen improves glycemic control in type1 diabetic animal model by promoting glucose uptake into skeletal muscle

https://www.ncbi.nlm.nih.gov/pmc/articles/PMC9889559/
(2023) Effectiveness and safety of hydrogen inhalation as an adjunct treatment in Chinese type 2 diabetes patients: A retrospective, observational, double-arm, real-life clinical study

https://www.ncbi.nlm.nih.gov/pmc/articles/PMC9515190/
Photocatalytic glucose depletion and hydrogen generation for diabetic wound healing

https://www.ncbi.nlm.nih.gov/pmc/articles/PMC7291681/
Molecular hydrogen improves type 2 diabetes through inhibiting oxidative stress

https://www.ncbi.nlm.nih.gov/pmc/articles/PMC5754517/
Subcutaneous injection of hydrogen gas is a novel effective treatment for type 2 diabetes

Eye Protection

https://pubmed.ncbi.nlm.nih.gov/19834032/
Protection of the retina by rapid diffusion of hydrogen: administration of hydrogen-loaded eye drops in retinal ischemia-reperfusion injury

https://pubmed.ncbi.nlm.nih.gov/20847117/
Hydrogen and N-acetyl-L-cysteine rescue oxidative stress-induced angiogenesis in a mouse corneal alkali-burn model

https://pubmed.ncbi.nlm.nih.gov/25801048/
Protective effect of molecular hydrogen against oxidative stress caused by peroxynitrite derived from nitric oxide in rat retina

Gut Health

https://www.ncbi.nlm.nih.gov/pmc/articles/PMC3231938/
Effects of drinking hydrogen-rich water on the quality of life of patients treated with radiotherapy for liver tumors

https://www.ncbi.nlm.nih.gov/pmc/articles/PMC3679390/
Hydrogen-rich water decreases serum LDL-cholesterol levels and improves HDL function in patients with potential metabolic syndrome

https://www.ncbi.nlm.nih.gov/pmc/articles/P

MC5799803/
Hydrogen-water ameliorates radiation-induced gastrointestinal toxicity via MyD88's effects on the gut microbiota

Hearing Loss

https://pubmed.ncbi.nlm.nih.gov/19339905/
Hydrogen protects auditory hair cells from free radicals

https://pubmed.ncbi.nlm.nih.gov/22387110/
Hydrogen-rich saline alleviates experimental noise-induced hearing loss in guinea pigs

https://www.ncbi.nlm.nih.gov/pmc/articles/PMC4063935/
Hydrogen-saturated saline protects intensive narrow band noise-induced hearing loss in guinea pigs through an antioxidant effect

Hormone Health

https://www.ncbi.nlm.nih.gov/pmc/articles/PMC6178641/
Emerging mechanisms and novel applications of hydrogen gas therapy

https://pubmed.ncbi.nlm.nih.gov/28560519/
Molecular hydrogen affects body composition, metabolic profiles, and mitochondrial function in middle-aged overweight women

https://www.ncbi.nlm.nih.gov/pmc/articles/P

MC10141176/
Therapeutic Potential of Molecular Hydrogen in Metabolic Diseases from Bench to Bedside

Hypertension

https://www.ncbi.nlm.nih.gov/pmc/articles/PMC9585236/
(2022) The effect of a low dose hydrogen-oxygen mixture inhalation in midlife/older adults with hypertension: A randomized, placebo-controlled trial

https://www.ncbi.nlm.nih.gov/pmc/articles/PMC7692487/
Daily inhalation of hydrogen gas has a blood pressure-lowering effect in a rat model of hypertension

https://pubmed.ncbi.nlm.nih.gov/30259991/
Hydrogen gas reduces chronic intermittent hypoxia-induced hypertension by inhibiting sympathetic nerve activity and increasing vasodilator responses via the antioxidation

Immune System

https://www.ncbi.nlm.nih.gov/pmc/articles/PMC7376192/
Hydrogen-rich water reduces inflammatory responses and prevents apoptosis of peripheral blood cells in healthy adults: a randomized, double-blind, controlled trial

https://www.ncbi.nlm.nih.gov/pmc/articles/PMC6567800/
Recent Advances in Studies of Molecular Hydrogen against Sepsis

https://www.ncbi.nlm.nih.gov/pmc/articles/PMC3560832/
Hydrogen-rich saline protects immunocytes from radiation-induced apoptosis

https://www.ncbi.nlm.nih.gov/pmc/articles/PMC7495244/
Hydrogen: A Novel Option in Human Disease Treatment

Liver Health

https://www.ncbi.nlm.nih.gov/pmc/articles/PMC5350887/
Effect of hydrogen-rich water on oxidative stress, liver function, and viral load in patients with chronic hepatitis B

https://pubmed.ncbi.nlm.nih.gov/23682614/
Effects of oral intake of hydrogen water on liver fibrogenesis in mice

https://www.ncbi.nlm.nih.gov/pmc/articles/PMC5350887/
Effect of hydrogen-rich water on oxidative stress, liver function, and viral load in patients with chronic hepatitis B

https://www.ncbi.nlm.nih.gov/pmc/articles/P

MC10196827/
A strategy of local hydrogen capture and catalytic hydrogenation for enhanced therapy of chronic liver diseases

https://www.ncbi.nlm.nih.gov/pmc/articles/PMC8002796/
Hydrogen treatment: a novel option in liver diseases

Metabolic / Weight Management

https://onlinelibrary.wiley.com/doi/10.1038/oby.2011.6
Molecular hydrogen improves obesity and diabetes by inducing hepatic FGF21 and stimulating energy metabolism in db/db mice

https://www.ncbi.nlm.nih.gov/pmc/articles/PMC9967957/
The Effects of Hydrogen-Rich Water on Blood Lipid Profiles in Clinical Populations: A Systematic Review and Meta-Analysis

https://www.ncbi.nlm.nih.gov/pmc/articles/PMC3679390/
Hydrogen-rich water decreases serum LDL-cholesterol levels and improves HDL function in patients with potential metabolic syndrome

Mood Disorders

https://www.ncbi.nlm.nih.gov/pmc/articles/PMC4812321/

Effects of hydrogen-rich water on depressive-like behavior in mice

https://www.ncbi.nlm.nih.gov/pmc/articles/PMC3409143/
Molecular Hydrogen Reduces LPS-Induced Neuroinflammation and Promotes Recovery from Sickness Behavior in Mice

https://www.ncbi.nlm.nih.gov/pmc/articles/PMC5575246/
Molecular hydrogen increases resilience to stress in mice

Parkinson's

https://hydrogenstudies.com/study/a-randomized-double-blind-multi-center-trial-of-hydrogen-water-for-parkinsons-disease-protocol-and-baseline-characteristics/
A randomized double-blind multi-center trial of hydrogen water for Parkinson's disease: protocol and baseline characteristics

https://bmcneurol.biomedcentral.com/articles/10.1186/s12883-016-0589-0
A randomized double-blind multi-center trial of hydrogen water for Parkinson's disease: protocol and baseline characteristics

https://www.sciencedirect.com/science/article/abs/pii/S0304394009001839?via%3Dihub
Molecular hydrogen is protective against 6-hydroxydopamine-induced nigrostriatal

degeneration in a rat model of Parkinson's disease

Safety / Tolerability

https://www.ncbi.nlm.nih.gov/pmc/articles/PMC5731988/
Molecular hydrogen: a preventive and therapeutic medical gas for various diseases

https://www.scientific.net/MSF.706-709.520
Influence of Hydrogen Discharged from Palladium Base Hydrogen Storage Alloys on Cancer Cells

https://www.sciencedirect.com/science/article/pii/S0163725814000941?via%3Dihub
Molecular hydrogen as a preventive and therapeutic medical gas: initiation, development and potential of hydrogen medicine

https://www.mdpi.com/2571-8797/2/4/33
Hydrogen Is Promising for Medical Applications

Skin Health

https://www.ncbi.nlm.nih.gov/pmc/articles/PMC3407032/
Hydrogen(H2) treatment for acute erythematous skin diseases. A report of 4 patients with safety data and a non-controlled feasibility study with H2

concentration measurement on two volunteers

https://www.ncbi.nlm.nih.gov/pmc/articles/PMC3852999/
The Drinking Effect of Hydrogen Water on Atopic Dermatitis Induced by Dermatophagoides farinae Allergen in NC/Nga Mice

Traumatic Brain Injury

https://www.ncbi.nlm.nih.gov/pmc/articles/PMC9224395/
Molecular Hydrogen Neuroprotection in Post-Ischemic Neurodegeneration in the Form of Alzheimer's Disease Proteinopathy: Underlying Mechanisms and Potential for Clinical Implementation—Fantasy or Reality?

https://www.tandfonline.com/doi/full/10.1080/01616412.2020.1747717
Hydrogen improves cell viability partly through inhibition of autophagy and activation of PI3K/Akt/GSK3β signal pathway in a microvascular endothelial cell model of traumatic brain injury

https://www.ijcep.com/files/ijcep0042919.pdf
Effect of hydrogen-rich water on the angiogenesis in lesion boundary brain tissue of traumatic brain injury-challenged rats

https://www.journalofsurgicalresearch.com/article/S0022-4804(18)30189-6/abstract
Hydrogen-rich water attenuates oxidative stress in rats with traumatic brain injury via Nrf2 pathway

Looking for more research? There are over 2,400 studies on H_2 and counting! To dive deeper, check out PubMed, Google Scholar, and the Molecular Hydrogen Institute for the latest findings. You can also visit HydroHeal.com and HydrogenStudies.com for additional resources. Pro tip: just type your condition + "molecular hydrogen" to quickly find relevant research.

Visit our website:

**MVTonline.com or
biohackingunlimited.com**

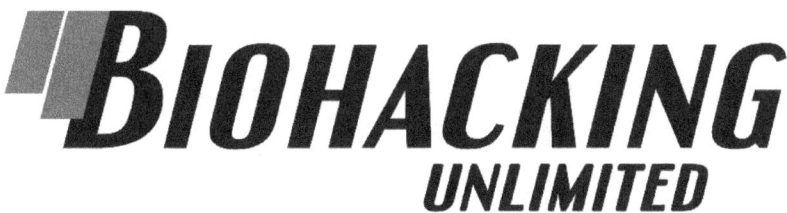

www.ingramcontent.com/pod-product-compliance
Lightning Source LLC
Chambersburg PA
CBHW052244220526
45471CB00001B/190

www.ingramcontent.com/pod-product-compliance
Lightning Source LLC
Chambersburg PA
CBHW052234220526
45471CB00001B/36